Long-term Care at Home Consumer Guide

WALTER FELDESMAN

Long-term Care at Home Consumer Guide

Introduction to Home Care
+
Where to Obtain Home Care
+
Original Medicare (Parts A/B)
+
Medicaid – A Federal and State Source of Payment
+
Original Medicare Outpatient Prescription Drugs (Part D)
+
Medicare Advantage Plans (MAP)
+
Medicare Advantage Outpatient Prescription Drugs (Part D)
+
Medicare Supplemental Insurance (Medigap)

Private Payment for Home Care
+
Long-term Care Insurance
+
Using a Home to Private Pay for Home Care
+
Private Pay with Life Insurance Accelerated Benefits
+
Use of Adult Day Care Centers for Eldercare Outside the Home
+
Use of Annuities to Private Pay for Eldercare
+
Alternative Housing Facilities
+
Federal Housing and Subsidies

©2009, by WALTER FELDESMAN

All rights reserved. No part of this book may be reproduced, stored in or introduced in a retrieval system, or transmitted in any form or by any means (electronic, mechanical, photocopying, recording or otherwise), without the prior written permission from the publisher, except for the inclusion of brief quotations in a review or for the private use of readers.

ISBN 978-0-578-01565-1

Publisher
Walter Feldesman
300 East 56th Street, 16-C
New York, NY 10022

NOTE:
The contents of this book is designed to provide information on the subjects it covers. It is published and/or otherwise disseminated with the understanding that neither the publisher nor any person or entity associated with him is engaged in rendering legal, accounting, or other professional services with respect to any of the subjects of the book. If legal or other expert assistance is required, the services of competent professional help should be sought. Although the publisher/author has made every effort to ensure the accuracy and completeness of information contained in the book, he assumes no responsibility for errors, inaccuracies, omissions, or inconsistencies.

To the memory of my dear wife, Lucille

✦

INTRODUCTION

Long-term Care at Home Consumer Guide

It is an established fact that chronically ill and disabled individuals, particularly the elderly, prefer to receive care at home rather than in an institution. The reason is simple. The family can provide care in the continued warmth and intimacy of the home. In addition, the family and home also offer a sense of independence, well-being, and undiminished quality of life.

Satisfying the preference for care at home does not come easily. When it comes to home care for their dear ones, families have a formidable task of navigating the intricacies of access to the health delivery system and the ways to pay for home care. Federal, state, and community programs and sources of information are fragmented and not easy to understand. Furthermore, from traditional Medicare to Medicaid, from services of the aging network to private Medicare Advantage plans, each program and funding source has its own complex requirements.

With *Long-term Care at Home Consumer Guide*, I have endeavored to compile and distill information about home care into a unique, user-friendly reference tool. I set two goals. The first is to create a product that offers one-stop-shopping for anyone needing to learn about caring for the elderly at home. The first goal contributes to the realization of the second: to develop a work that facilitates a family solution to long-term care at home, rather than in an institution, for chronically ill and disabled older Americans.

The *Guide* addresses three basic questions. **What is home care? Where and how can it be obtained? What are the sources for paying for it?** The elusive answers to these common questions are necessary for average consumers and useful and convenient for eldercare professionals such as geriatric care managers, private and public agency personnel assisting seniors, attorneys, and individuals in the various health care fields, and, most particularly, for the elderly and their families.

The *Guide* gathers the most up-to-date information across a comprehensive array of eldercare topics. It is an outgrowth of my two previous publications –

Dictionary of Eldercare Terminology (2nd edition, 2000) and *Long-term Care at Home: The Family Solution* (2001), both published by the National Information Services Corporation (NISC).

In addition to this print version of the *Long-term Care at Home Consumer Guide,* it also is published in a web-based electronic format which is available at *www.biblioline.com/eldercare/consumer*. Compared to a traditional printed book, the electronic publication offers considerable advantages, especially the capability of searching the contents of the volume by topic or key word. Electronic searching is speedier, less cumbersome and more convenient than the multiple searching for information in a conventional book.

Specialists or consumers seeking information in greater depth than found in the *Guide* can consult the four volumes of my *Eldercare Primer + Series*:

Volume I, *Original Medicare Program*
Volume II, *Medicare Advantage Program*
Volume III, *Federal Entitlements*
Volume IV, *Private Payment for Eldercare and Housing.*

These four volumes are being published simultaneously with the *Guide*. Electronic copies can be found on-line at *www.biblioline.com/eldercare.*

-- Walter Feldesman, J.D.
Harvard

USING *LONG-TERM CARE AT HOME CONSUMER GUIDE*

To help readers search for specific information in the *Guide*, it employs several devices. First, it is laid out in a **question-and-answer format**; it poses most of the frequently asked questions about home care and provides authoritative answers. Second, within the text, **key terms and concepts** appear in bold type, and critical points are underlined or set in bold type.

The *Guide* incorporates other user-friendly features:

- A detailed **Table of Contents** sets forth, by section and subsection, each Chapter's subject matter. The Table of Contents presents the substance of the entire *Guide* in an outline format.

- **Topical Indices (TI)** for most chapters break down the subject matter of a particular Chapter into key points and topics.

- A comprehensive **Word Index (WI)** sets forth the salient words and terms found throughout the text.

The *Guide* is also available on-line in an electronic format. Visit *www.biblioline.com/eldercare/consumer*.

NAVIGATING THE ON-LINE VERSION OF
Long-term Care at Home Consumer Guide

For the convenience of readers, the *Long-term Care at Home Consumer Guide* is organized in an outline format and according to the questions that consumers are likely to pose about long-term care for their loved ones at home.

A detailed Table of Contents reflects the major sections and subsections of the outline. Within the text, key terms appear in bold type, and critical points are underlined or set in bold type.

The *Guide* can be downloaded and searched without charge. According to the copyright restrictions set by the author, **only limited portions of the book may be printed** by users.

The *Guide* can be searched electronically in two ways. First, readers can use the features of BiblioLine℠ which are explained in detail at *www.biblioline.com/eldercare/consumer*. Or readers can utilize the search features of Adobe Acrobat Reader which are explained in the following pages. A free download of the latest version of Acrobat Reader (9.0) is available at *www.adobe.com/products/acrobat/readstep2.html* or by clicking this icon In order to take advantage of Adobe Acrobat Reader's convenient search features, users of the *Guide* must employ version 9.0 or higher.

Use of On-line Version

To download the *Guide*, click on the title that appears on the *Guide*'s home page. This will lead to the page shown below:

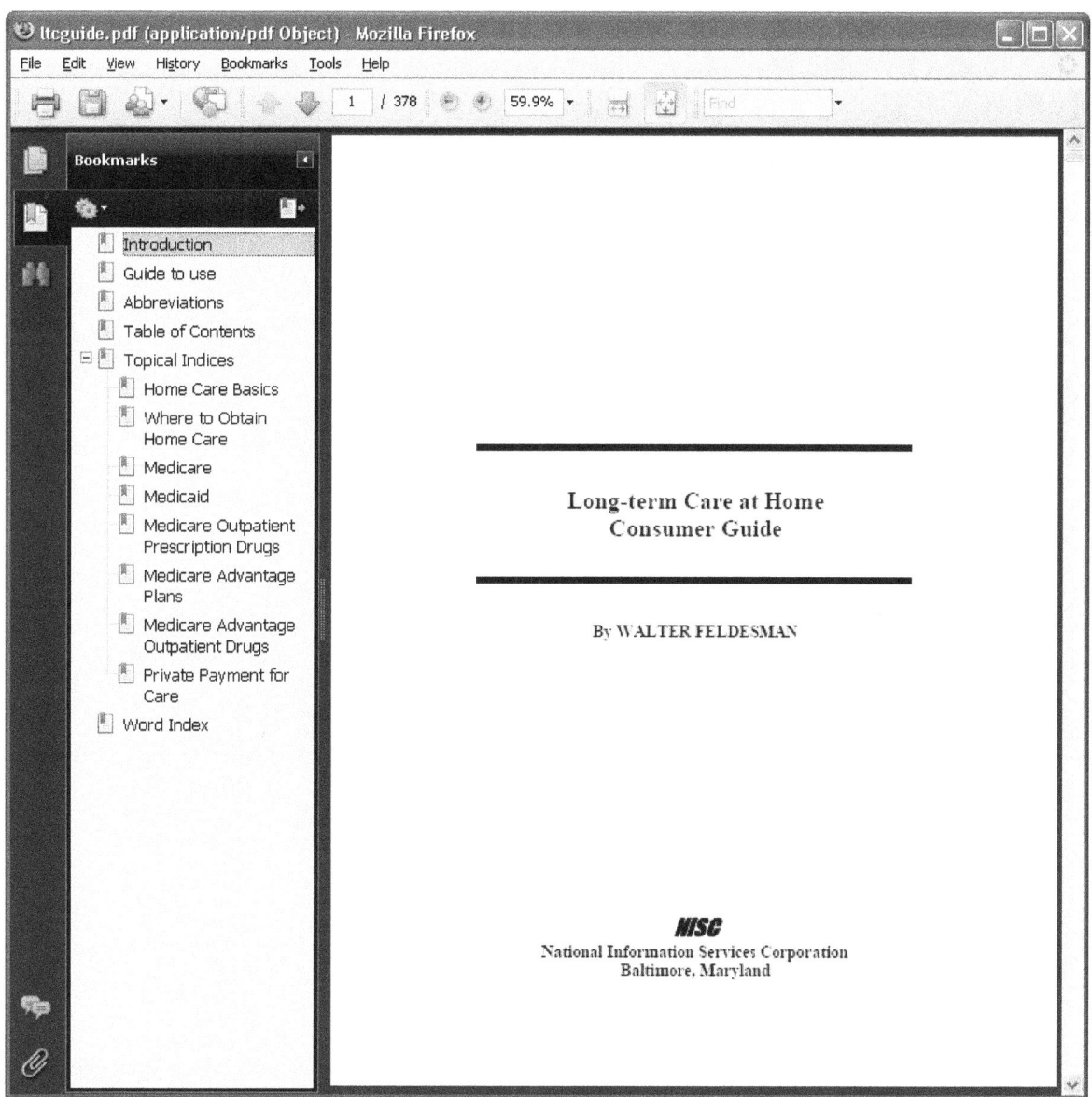

The bookmarks in the left-hand column are hot linked and will go to each major section of the *Guide*.

The quickest way to obtain an overview of the *Guide* and to navigate to a specific topic is to proceed to the Table of Contents shown on the following page.

Use of On-line Version
(continued)

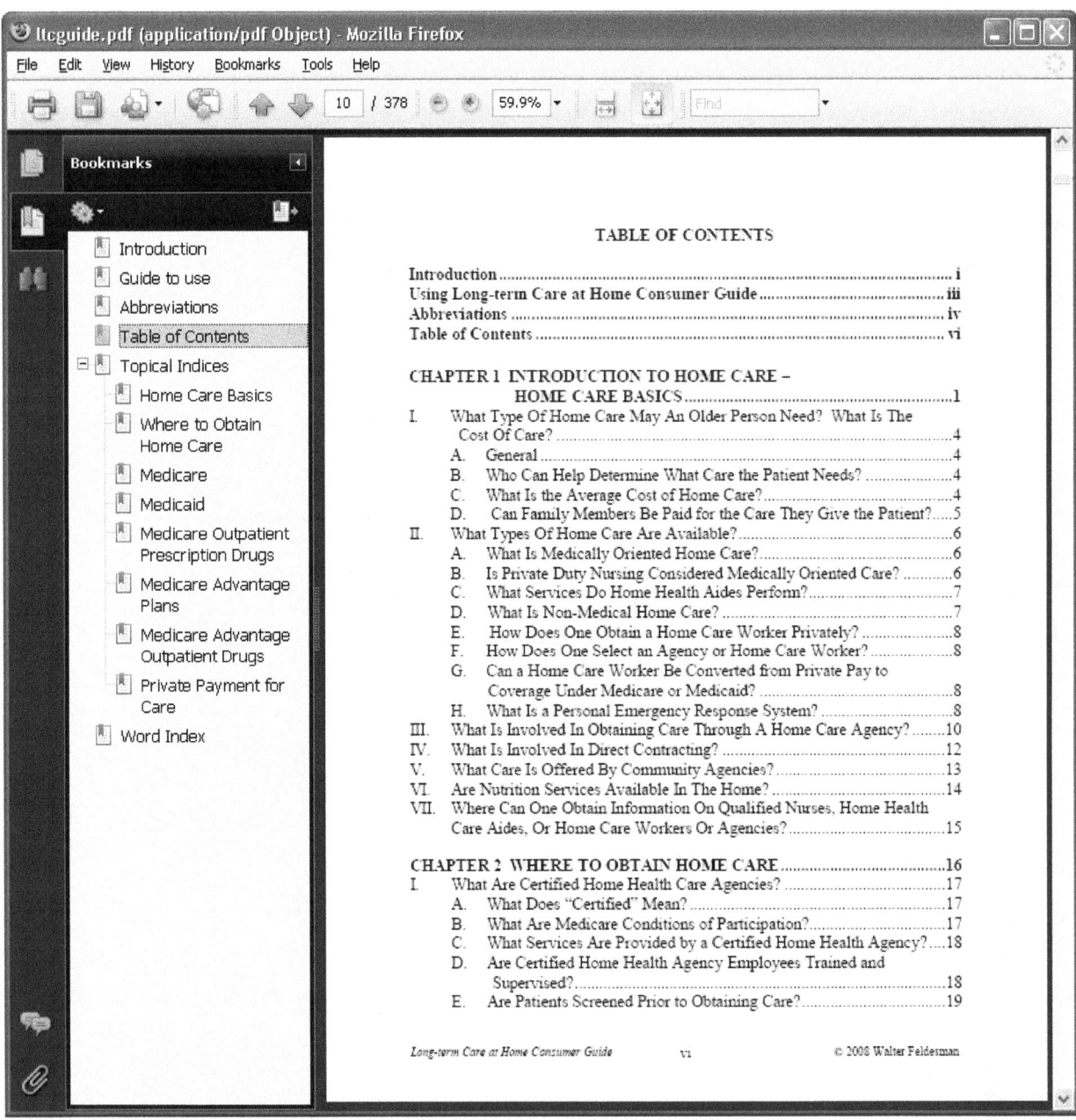

Each topic and question in the Table of Contents is hot linked. **Clicking on the page numbers in the right-hand column** will lead directly to the relevant topic or question in the *Guide*.

Use of On-line Version (continued)

To Search the *Guide*

A search for specific information in the *Guide* can be accomplished in two ways. First, readers may consult the two indices – one of words and the other of topics – that appear at the end of the *Guide*. Page numbers listed in the indices are hot linked so that readers are taken directly to the relevant page.

Second, an electronic search of the *Guide* is possible by using the search feature available in version 9.0 or higher of Adobe Acrobat Reader. (See above for information about how to download the most current version of this program without cost.)

To activate a search, click on the binocular icon on the extreme right-hand side of the screen. This will lead to a search column shown below:

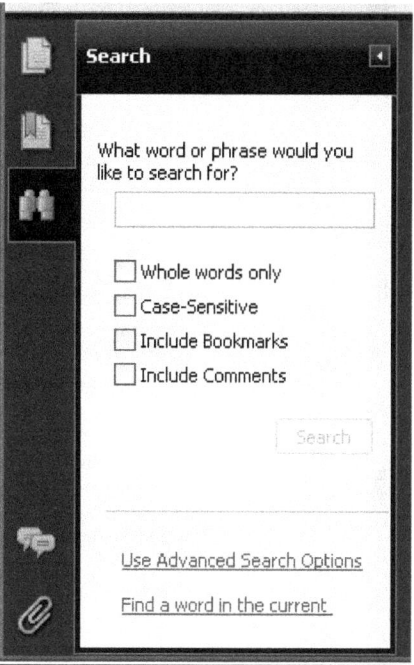

A search for a specific word/term or combination of words found in the *Guide* is possible. The word or term is highlighted in the text as show in the following page.

Use of On-line Version
(continued)

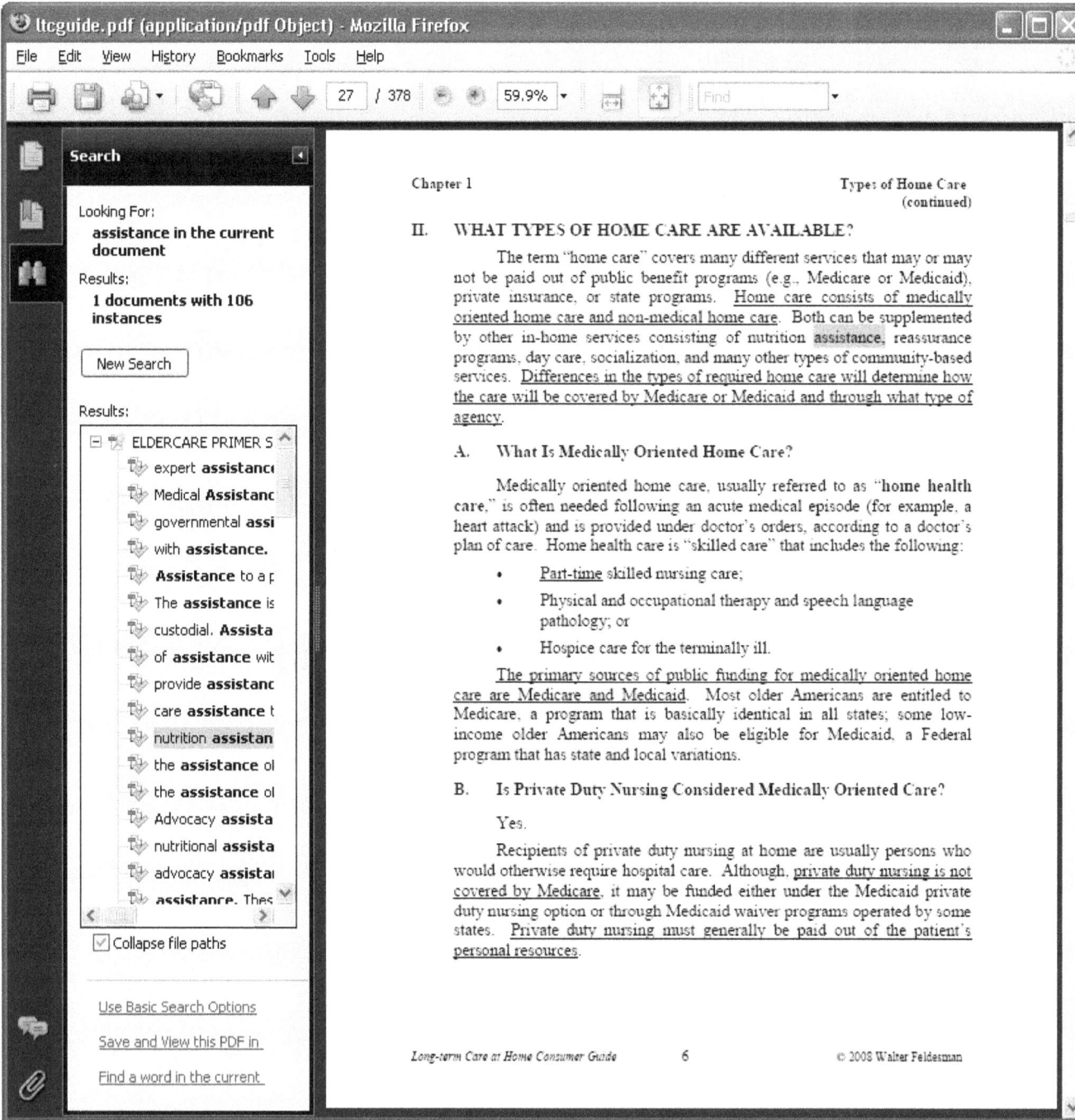

Long-term Care at Home Consumer Guide   viii   © 2009 Walter Feldesman

ABBREVIATIONS & ACRONYMS

AAA	Area Agency on Aging
ADL	Activity of daily living
ALJ	Administrative law judge
AoA	Administration on Aging
BBA	Balanced Budget Act
CHHA	Certified home health agency
CCRC	Continuing care retirement community
CMS	Centers for Medicare and Medicaid Services
COBRA	Consolidated Omnibus Budget Reconciliation Act
DAB	Departmental appeals board
DME	Durable medical equipment
ESRD	End-stage renal disease
FFS	Fee-for-service
HCFA	Health Care Financing Administration (see also CMS)
HDHP	High-deductible health policy
HHA	Home health agency
HHS	Health and Human Services, U. S. Department of
HIPAA	Health Insurance Portability and Accountability Act of 1996
HMO	Health maintenance organization
HUD	Housing and Urban Development, U.S. Department of
IADL	Instrumental activities of daily living
IRE	Independent review entity
LTC	Long-term care
LTCI	Long-term care insurance

MA	Medicare Advantage (formerly Medicare + Choice)
MA-PDP	Medicare Advantage Prescription Drug Plan
MMA	Medicare Prescription Drug, Improvement, and Modernization Act of 2003
MSA	Medical savings account
OAA	Older Americans Act
OBRA	Omnibus Budget Reconciliation Act
PACE	Program for all-inclusive care of the elderly
PCP	Primary care physician
PDP	Prescription drug plan
PFFS	Private fee-for-service
PHA	Public housing agency
POS	Point of service
PPO	Preferred provider organization
PSO	Provider-sponsored organization
QDWI	Qualified disabled and working individual
QI-1	Qualifying individual
QIC	Qualified independent contractor
QIO	Quality improvement organization
QMB	Qualified Medicare beneficiary
RFB	Religious fraternal benefits (coordinated care plan)
SLMB	Specified low-income Medicare beneficiary
SNF	Skilled nursing facility
SNP	Special needs plan
SSA	Social Security Administration
SSI	Supplemental Security Income

SUA   State unit on aging

TEFRA   Tax Equity and Fiscal Responsibility Act

TABLE OF CONTENTS

Introduction i
Using Long-term Care at Home Consumer Guide iii
Navigating the On-line Edition iv
Abbreviations and Acronyms ix
Table of Contents xiii

**CHAPTER 1 INTRODUCTION TO HOME CARE –
HOME CARE BASICS** 1

I. What Type of Home Care May an Older Person Need? What Is the
 Cost of Care? 4
 A. General 4
 B. Who Can Help Determine What Care the Patient Needs? 4
 C. What Is the Average Cost of Home Care? 4
 D. Can Family Members Be Paid for the Care They Give the
 Patient? 5
II. What Types of Home Care Are Available? 6
 A. What Is Medically Oriented Home Care? 6
 B. Is Private Duty Nursing Considered Medically Oriented Care? 6
 C. What Services Do Home Health Aides Perform? 7
 D. What Is Non-medical Home Care? 7
 E. How Does One Obtain a Home Care Worker Privately? 8
 F. How Does One Select an Agency or Home Care Worker? 8
 G. Can a Home Care Worker Be Converted from Private Pay to
 Coverage under Medicare or Medicaid? 8
 H. What Is a Personal Emergency Response System? 8
III. What Is Involved in Obtaining Care Through a Home Care Agency? 10
IV. What Is Involved in Direct Contracting? 12
V. What Care Is Offered by Community Agencies? 13
VI. Are Nutrition Services Available in the Home? 14
VII. Where Can One Obtain Information on Qualified Nurses, Home Health
 Care Aides, or Home Care Workers or Agencies? 15

CHAPTER 2 WHERE TO OBTAIN HOME CARE 17
I. What Are Certified Home Health Care Agencies? 18
 A. What Does "Certified" Mean? 18
 B. What Are Medicare Conditions of Participation? 18
 C. What Services Are Provided by a Certified Home Health Agency? ... 19

	D.	Are Certified Home Health Agency Employees Trained and Supervised? 19
	E.	Are Patients Screened Prior to Obtaining Care? 20
	F.	What Are the Rights of Certified Home Health Agency Patients? 20
II.	What Are Licensed Home Care Agencies and Their Services? 22
	A.	What Services Are Provided by Licensed Home Care Agencies? 22
	B.	Who Uses the Services of Licensed Home Care Agencies? 22
	C.	What Happens When a Patient Depletes His/Her Own Resources? 23
III.	What Are Community-based Agencies and Their Services? 24
	A.	What Services May Be Available from Community Agencies? 24
IV.	What Are Adult Day Care Programs, Their Functions, and Fees? 25
	A.	What Are Adult Day Care Programs? 25
	B.	Who Are the Main Sources Providing Adult Day Care? 25
	C.	What Are the Different Levels of Adult Day Care? 26
	D.	Are There Fees for Adult Day Care? 27
	E.	Can Homebound Individuals Receiving Medicare Home Care Coverage Attend Adult Day Care Programs? 27
V.	What Are Area Agencies on Aging and Their Services? 28
	A.	Who Is Eligible for Services from an Area Agency on Aging? 28
	B.	Does Eligibility for Services Depend on Financial Need? 28
	C.	What Services Are Offered by an Area Agency on Aging? 28

CHAPTER 3 ORIGINAL MEDICARE (PARTS A/B) A FEDERAL SOURCE OF PAYMENT 31

I.	What Are the Eligibility Requirements for Medicare? 34
	A.	Who Is Eligible for Medicare Part A? 34
	B.	Who Is Eligible for Medicare Part B? 35
	C.	What Happens When People Cannot Afford Monthly Premiums? 36
	D.	Can People Have Both Medicare and Medicaid? 36
	E.	Can People Have Both Medicare and Employer-paid Health Insurance? 36
II.	What Are the Medicare Enrollment Requirements and Procedures? 37
	A.	How Does One Enroll in Medicare? 37
	B.	Who Is Eligible for Automatic Enrollment? 37
	C.	Who Has to Apply Separately to Enroll? 38
	D.	When Are the Enrollment Periods? 38
	E.	What Happens If an Application Is Not Filed on Time? 40
III.	What Are the Requirements for Medicare-covered Home Health Care? 41
	A.	How Does One Qualify for Medicare-covered Home Health Care? ... 41
	B.	What Are the Five Medicare Qualifying Conditions? 41

		C. What Are the Dependent Services? 44

- C. What Are the Dependent Services? 44
- D. What Types of Home Care Services Are Not Covered by Medicare? 49
- E. Are There Out-of-Pocket Costs When Receiving Medicare Home Care? 49

IV. What Is Hospice Care, and What Does Medicare Cover? 51
  - A. Who Is Eligible for Hospice Care? 51
  - B. What Are the Qualifying Conditions for Medicare Hospice Care? 51
  - C. What Services Are Included in Medicare Hospice Care? 52

V. What Is the Appeal Process for Home Care Denials, Reductions, or Termination of Services? 54
  - A. What Are the Steps Prior to an Appeal? 54
  - B. Can a Patient Appeal an Advance Notice to the Beneficiary from the Home Care Agency? 55
  - C. What Is the Medicare Part A and Part B Appeals Process of Home Health Claims? 56

VI. When Does Medicare Consider It Is a Secondary Payer and Another Plan Covering the Medicare Beneficiary Is the Primary Payer? 60

VII. What Is the Program for All-inclusive Home Care of the Elderly (PACE)? 60

VIII. Can a Physician Opt Out of Medicare? 62

IX. Is There Any Coordination of Coverage Between Medicare and Employer Plans? 63
  - A. What Is the Coverage Coordination for Employees Age 65 or Older? 63
  - B. What Is the Coverage Coordination for Retired Medicare-eligible Employees? 63

X. May Employees, When Their Employment Is Terminated, Have Continuing Medical Services Under Their Previous Employer's Medical Insurance Plan? 64

XI. Will Medicare Help Pay for Other Services Incidental to or Supplemental to Home Care? 65
  - A. What Are the Covered Outpatient Services? 65
  - B. For Which Outpatient Services Will Medicare Part B Not Pay? 69
  - C. Are There Cost-sharing Expenses, Deductibles, Premiums, Coinsurance for Part B Services? 71
  - D. What Is the Billing and Payment Process for Part B Services and Supplies? 72
  - E. Are There Special Rates for the Payment of Part B Services and Supplies to Low-income Beneficiaries? 73

APPENDIX A OUTPATIENT SKILLED THERAPY 77

I.	Homebound Not a Requirement	77
II.	Reasonable and Necessary Requirement	77
III.	Physician's Care Plan and Certification	78
IV.	Applicable Standards	78
V.	Amount of Payment by Patient	78
VI.	Financial Limitations (CAP)	79
VII.	Types of Therapists	79

APPENDIX B   OUTPATIENT DEPARTMENT HOSPITAL SERVICES ... 81

APPENDIX C   MENTAL HEALTH SERVICES FURNISHED BY HOSPITAL OUTPATIENT UNITS AND QUALIFIED COMMUNITY MENTAL HEALTH CENTERS 82

APPENDIX D   DURABLE MEDICAL EQUIPMENT 83

I.	Definition of Durable Medical Equipment	83
	A. Durability	83
	B. Medical Equipment.	83
II.	Requirements for Coverage	83
	A. Use in Patient's Home.	83
	B. Necessary and Reasonable.	84
	C. Prescription.	84
	D. Certificate of Medical Necessity (CMN).	84
III.	Repairs, Maintenance, Replacement and Delivery.	84
	A. Repairs.	84
	B. Maintenance.	84
	C. Replacement.	84
	D. Delivery.	84
IV.	Supplies and Accessories	85
V.	Oxygen Services in the Home	85
VI.	Purchase Option for Capped Rental Items.	85
VII.	Prosthetic Devices (Other than Dental)	85
	A. Examples of Prosthetic Devices.	85
	B. Prosthetic Lenses.	85
	C. Dentures.	86
	D. Supplies, Repairs, Adjustments, and Replacements.	86

APPENDIX E   AMBULANCE TRANSPORTATION 87

APPENDIX F   PREVENTIVE DISEASE MANAGEMENT SERVICES 88

I.	Annual Prostate Cancer Screening Tests	88
II.	Screening Pap Smears, Screening Pelvic Exam	88
III.	Screening Mammography	88
IV.	Cardiovascular Screening Blood Tests	88
V.	Diabetes Screenings	89

VI.	Colorectal Cancer Screening Tests: Fecal-Occult Blood Test, Flexible Sigmoidoscopy and Colonoscopy.	89
VII.	Glaucoma Screening	89
VIII.	Ultrasound Screening for Abdominal Aorta Aneurism	90
IX.	Preventive Physicals	90

APPENDIX G PRIVATE CONTRACTS **91**

I.	Beneficiary Protections	91
II.	No Limiting Charges	91
III.	Physician's or Practitioner's Required Affidavit	91

APPENDIX H COORDINATION OF COVERAGE – MEDICARE AND EMPLOYER PLANS **93**

I.	Carve-out Coverage.	93
II.	Wrap-around Coverage.	93
III.	Coordination of Benefits Coverage.	93
IV.	Exclusion Coverage.	93

CHAPTER 4 MEDICAID - A FEDERAL AND STATE SOURCE OF PAYMENT **95**

I.	What Are the Eligibility Criteria for Medicaid?		98
	A.	What Are the Factors to Establish Medicaid Eligibility?	98
	B.	What Are the Status Standards?	98
	C.	What Are the Income Standards?	98
	D.	What Are the Resource Standards?	99
	E.	Are the Income and Resource Eligibility Standards Which Apply to Single Individuals Applicable to Married Couples?	100
	F.	What Are the Categories of Eligibility?	106
	G.	According to Medicaid Trust Eligibility Rules, Is the Principal or the Income of Trusts Created by the Applicant Considered Countable Resources or Countable Income?	111
	H.	What Are Some Other State Eligibility Standards?	114
II.	What Are the Penalty Rules for the Transfer of Assets?		115
	A.	Can One Transfer Assets or Property to Become Medicaid-Eligible?	115
	B.	What Is a Look-back Period?	115
	C.	What Is a Prohibited Transfer of Assets?	117
	D.	What Is the Penalty for Making a Prohibited Transfer of Assets?	118
	E.	What Is the Period of Ineligibility?	118
	F.	Are Any Transfers Not Subject to a Penalty?	119
	G.	Are Transfers to or by a Trust Subject to the Trust Transfer Penalty Rules?	119

	H.	Is the Transfer Penalty Applicable to All Medicaid Services? 121
III.	Does Medicaid Offer Home Care Services to Medicaid Eligibles? 122
	A.	What Medicaid Services Are Federally Required? 122
	B.	What Medicaid Home Care Benefits Are Optional to States? 122
	C.	Which Home and Community-based Long-term Care Services Can a State Offer on a Waivered Basis? 122
	D.	What Is "Personal" Care Under Medicaid? 123
	E.	Are Personal Care Aides Trained and Supervised? 123
	F.	Are There Medicaid Qualifying Conditions for Home Health Care? 124
	G.	Does Medicaid Impose Qualifying Conditions for Personal Care Services? 124
	H.	How Does One Find Out about Individual State Programs? 125
IV.	Can Medicaid Recover Costs of Medical Assistance? 127
V.	What Are the Due Process Rights for Appealing Medicaid Decisions? 129
VI.	Can Medicaid Mandate Managed Care? 130
	A.	Is Anyone Eligible for Medicaid Exempt from Mandatory Enrollment in Managed Care? 130
	B.	Does an Individual Have a Choice of Managed Care Entities? 130
	C.	Are Medicaid Recipients Guaranteed Eligibility to a Managed Care Entity? 130
	D.	What Are an Individual's Rights When Terminating or Changing Enrollment in a Medicaid Managed Care Organization? 131
	E.	What Information Must Be Provided to a Medicaid Managed Care Participant? 131
	F.	What Access to Emergency Services Do Medicaid Managed Care Participants Have? 131
	G.	Can a Medicare Managed Care Organization Restrict Enrollee-Provider Communications? 132
	H.	How Are Medicaid Managed Care Organization and Primary Care Case Management Defined? 132
VII.	Can State Long-term Partnership Programs Affect Medicaid Income and/or Resource Eligibility Standards? 134
	A.	What Are the Requirements of a Qualified State Long-term Care Insurance Policy? 135

CHAPTER 5 ORIGINAL MEDICARE PRESCRIPTION DRUGS (PART D) 137

I.	What Is the Medicare Prescription Drug Program? 137
II.	What Is a Part D Drug Under the Medicare Part D Program? 139

III. Who Is Eligible to Enroll in the Part D Prescription Drug Program, and When Can an Individual Eligible for Part D Enroll? 140
   A. Who Is Eligible? 140
   B. In Order to Obtain Part D Drugs, Is It Necessary to Enroll In A Prescription Drug Plan? 140
   C. When Are the Periods to Enroll for Medicare Part D Coverage? 141
   D. What Is the Effective Date of Enrollment Coverage? 142
   E. Can an Enrollee of a Prescription Drug Plan Change Plans Mid-Year? 143
   F. Is There a Penalty for Late Enrollment? 143
IV. What Are the Costs of the Prescription Drug Plans? 145
   A. What Are the Costs of the Standard Drug Plan? 145
   B. What Are the Costs of an Alternative Prescription Drug Coverage Plan? 146
   C. Are Subsidies Available to Help Low-income Individuals Pay for Part D Drug Coverage? 147
V. How Does a Person Eligible for Part D Join a PDP? 149
VI. Are the Costs of Prescription Drugs Under Prescription Drug Plans Less for Low-income Individuals? 151
   A. Who Are the Low-income Beneficiaries? 151
   B. What Part D Drug Subsidies Are Provided to Low-income Individuals? 152

CHAPTER 6 MEDICARE ADVANTAGE PLANS (MAP) A FEDERAL SOURCE OF PAYMENT 155

I. What Are Medicare Advantage Plans? 155
II. What Features Are Common to Medicare Advantage Plans? 157
   A. What Are the Types of Medicare Advantage Plans? 157
   B. Do MAPs Have a Minimum Enrollment Requirement? 158
   C. How Does a Beneficiary Enroll or Disenroll in a MAP? 158
   D. What Are the Enrollment Periods? 158
   E. What Are the Premiums for MAPs? 161
   F. Are There Limits on Enrollee Cost-sharing? 161
   G. What Are the Basic, Additional and Supplemental Benefits of MAPs? 162
   H. To What Services Does an Enrollee Have Access in Medicare Advantage Coordinated Care Plans and Network MSA Plans? 163
   I. How Does Medicare Treat Payments to Medicare Advantage Organizations? 164
   J. What Emergency Services Must a Medicare Advantage Plan Provide? . 164

K. In Which Instances May a Medicare Advantage Organization Balance Bill or Not? 165
L. Must a MA Plan Offer Part D Drug Coverage? 166
M. What Is the Appeal Process for Home Care Denials, Reductions or Termination of Services? 166

Appendix A Grievances – Organization Determinations, Reconsiderations and Appeals 167

Appendix B Fast-Track Appeals to the Independent Review Entity 177

III. What Special Features Do the Different Medicare Advantage Plans Have? 179

Appendix C   Coordinated Care Plans (CCP) 180
Appendix C-1 HMO Plans 183
Appendix C-2 Preferred Provider Organization (PPO) Plans 185
Appendix C-3 Provider-sponsored Organization (PSO) Plans 189
Appendix C-4 Religious Fraternal Benefits (RFB) Plans 191
Appendix C-5 Specialized Medicare Advantage Plans for Special Needs Beneficiaries (SNP) 193
APPENDIX D Medical Savings Account (MSA) Plans 196
APPENDIX E Private Fee-for-Service (PFFS) Plan 204

CHAPTER 7 MEDICARE ADVANTAGE OUTPATIENT PRESCRIPTION DRUG PLANS (MA – PDP) 207

I. What Are MA Prescription Drug Plans? 207
   A. What Are Part D Drugs? 207
   B. What Is Included in a MA-PDP Drug Formulary? 207
   C. May Medigap Policies Include Drug Coverage? 208
   D. Can Medicare Negotiate Drug Discounts? 208
   E. Does Medicaid Cover Part D Drugs? 208
   F. How Much Cost-sharing Is There for Part D Drug Coverage? 208
   G. Is a Subsidy Program Available? 211
   H. Are Persons with End-stage Renal Disease Eligible for Part D Benefits? 211
II. How Does One Enroll in a Medicare Advantage Prescription Drug Plan? 212
   A. Does Participation in a Medicare Advantage Plan Require Enrollment in its Prescription Drug Plan? 212
   B. What Are the Enrollment Periods? 213
   C. When Can a Beneficiary Change Plans? 215
   D. What Happens If a Beneficiary Fails to Enroll on a Timely Basis? .. 216

      E.   What Is the Enrollment Process for Individuals Who Are Full-benefit Dual Eligible? 216
III.   Are Subsidies Available for Low-income Individuals? 218
      A.   Who Are the Subsidy-eligible Individuals? 218
      B.   How Much Are the Premium Subsidies? 219
      C.   How Much Are the Subsidies for Drug Cost-sharing? 220

CHAPTER 8 MEDICARE SUPPLEMENTAL INSURANCE (MEDIGAP) 223

I.   What Is Medigap Insurance? 225
II.   What Are the Key Characteristics of Medigap Polices? 225
III.   What Are the Benefit Packages of the Medigap Plans? 227
IV.   What Are Plans K and L? 228
V.   Do Medigap Policies Cover Prescription Drugs? 229
VI.   What Are Medigap High-deductible Policies? 229
VII. What Is a Medicare Select Policy? 229
VIII. Do Any Medigap Policies Cover Home Care? 230
IX.   Is There an Exclusion (Waiting or Elimination) Period Due to a Pre-existing Medical Condition? 230
X.   Are Individuals Guaranteed Issue of Plans A, B, C and F Despite a Pre-existing Medical Condition? 231
XI.   Summary of Medigap Benefits 233

CHAPTER 9 PRIVATE LONG-TERM CARE INSURANCE 235

I.   What Is Long-term Care Insurance? 237
II.   What Is a Classic Long-term Care Policy? 237
III.   What Is an Integrated Long-term Care Policy? 237
IV.   What Are Some of the Key Characteristics of Long-term Care Insurance? 237
V.   What Are Trigger Events? 238
VI.   What Is the Cost of Long-term Care Insurance? 239
VII. Is There a Penalty for Non-payment of Premiums? 240
VIII. What Are the Benefits of Long-term Care Insurance? 240
IX.   Do Long-term Care Policies Include a Deductible Before Payments Begin? 241
X.   Can One Buy a Long-term Care Policy When There Is a Pre-existing Condition? 242
XI.   Can One Upgrade a Long-term Care Insurance Policy? 242
XII. What Is the Benefit of a Non-forfeiture Clause? 242
XIII. Can One Reinstate a Policy After It Unintentionally Lapses? 243

XIV. What Are the Requirements for a Policy to Be Tax-qualified? 243
XV. What Conditions Must Be Met to Obtain Tax-qualified Benefits? 243
XVI. What Are the Tax Advantages of a Tax-qualified LTCI Policy? 245
XVII. What Are State Partnership Programs For LTCI (Robert Wood Johnson Programs)? 246
XVIII. Can One Obtain More Information About Long-term Care Insurance? ... 246

CHAPTER 10 PRIVATE PAYMENT FOR HOME CARE 247
I. What Is Direct Contracting? 247
II. What Are the Advantages of Using a Home Health Agency? 248
III. How Can the Services of a Geriatric Care Manager Be Useful? 249

CHAPTER 11 USING A HOME TO PAY FOR HOME CARE 251
I. What Are Home Equity Conversion Plans? 251
II. What Is a Residential Sale-Leaseback? 251
III. What Is a Reverse Mortgage? 251
IV. Who Can Obtain a Reverse Mortgage? 252
V. What Is the Effect of a Reverse Mortgage on Medicaid Eligibility? 253
VI. Can Lenders and Home Owners Be Insured Against Default and Eviction? 253
VII. Do State Laws Regulate Reverse Mortgages? 254

CHAPTER 12 ACCELERATED BENEFITS OF A LIFE INSURANCE POLICY TO PAY FOR HOME CARE 255
I. How Can One Use a Life Insurance Policy for Home Care? 255
II. Are There Tax Advantages for Using Life Insurance During One's Lifetime? 256
III. What Are the Conditions for a Chronically Ill Individual to Obtain Tax Advantages for Accelerated Benefits? 256
IV. What Are the Tax Advantages of Accelerated Living Benefits to a Chronically Ill Individual? 257
V. How Does One Obtain Accelerated Living Benefits? 257
VI. Do Living Benefits from a Life Insurance Policy Affect Medicaid Eligibility? 257
VII. Who Is a Viatical Provider? 258
VIII. Where Does One Obtain Information on These Various Options? 258

CHAPTER 13 USE OF ADULT DAY CARE CENTERS FOR ELDERCARE OUTSIDE THE HOME 259
I. What Are Adult Day Care Centers? 259
II. What Are the Fees for Services? 260

III. How Does Attendance at an Adult Day Care Center Effect One's Homebound Status?.. 260

CHAPTER 14 USE OF ANNUITIES TO PAY FOR ELDERCARE........... 261
I. What Are the Types of Annuities? 261
II. What Is the Tax Treatment of Annuities?..................................... 262

CHAPTER 15 ALTERNATIVE HOUSING FACILITIES –
 PRIVATE PAYMENT 263
I. What Institutional, Non-medical Facilities Are Available for Dependent Residents?.. 263
II. What Non-institutional, Non-medical Facilities Are Available for Semi-dependent Residents? 264
III. What Non-institutional, Non-medical Facilities Are Available for Independent Residents?... 265
IV. What Other Alternative Housing Arrangements Are Available?............... 267

CHAPTER 16 FEDERAL HOUSING AND SUBSIDIES 271
I. What Are the Most Frequently Used Federal Housing Subsidy Housing Programs? 271
　A. What Is the Section 8 Rental Subsidy Program (Voucher Program)?271
　B. What Is the Section 202 Program of Supportive Housing for the Elderly? 273
　C. What Is the Congregate Housing Services Program? 274

TOPICAL INDICES...275
　Home Care Basics.. 275
　Where to Obtain Home Care.. 279
　Medicare 281
　Medicaid 291
　Medicare Outpatient Prescription Drugs 301
　Medicare Advantage Plans 307
　Medicare Advantage Outpatient Drugs 317
　Private Payment for Care 321

WORD INDEX..327

CHAPTER 1

INTRODUCTION TO HOME CARE – HOME CARE BASICS

Home care services permit an impaired older person to live at home independently, in a familiar environment, rather than in the institutional setting of a nursing home, or in a board-and-care facility. **As a general rule, any person who is not acutely ill can be adequately cared for in the home** provided his/her resources, governmental assistance and/or community-based services are available. The home care package needed by each individual depends on idiosyncratic factors reflecting the individual's personal, social, familial, and financial circumstances, as well as the individual's medical diagnosis, prognosis, mental condition, and the ability to function at home with assistance.

An organized home care program can be provided through a combination of: (i) **informal caregivers**, especially family members; (ii) **formal caregivers** who are medical or other trained persons, such as doctors, nurses, home health aides, therapists, geriatric care managers and social workers; and (iii) **non-medical persons**, such as personal care aides, homemakers, community volunteers and city or state personnel. Under the direction of a physician, the care can be oriented to a patient's needs. It may be similar to the level of **skilled care** provided in a skilled nursing facility (e.g., nursing nutritional services, physical, occupational and speech therapy), and more often than not it can be unskilled care in the nature of **custodial** or **personal care**.

Family members and friends are the largest single source of support and care for older persons who continue to live at home, but are limited in one or more **activities of daily living (ADL)**. ADLs consist of activities usually performed for oneself in the course of a normal day and are usually considered to be **mobility** (e.g., transfer from, or to a bed or chair), **dressing**, **bathing**, **eating** and **toileting**. Assistance to a person limited in his or her ADLs is customarily performed by a family member, home health aide or attendant (or a nurse's aide in a nursing facility). **The assistance is of a non-medical nature (physical) commonly characterized as personal care, or custodial.** Assistance provided in a home setting goes beyond ADLs to non-medical activities commonly referred to as **instrumental activities of daily living (IADL).** These include **housekeeping** and **homemaker's chores** (e.g., cleaning, cooking, laundry and shopping). **Medicare cannot be looked to for payment of services, except to a limited extent if and when related to dependent services (described in Chapter 3 section III.C), for coverage of assistance with ADLs or IADLs.**

Chapter 1   Introduction to Home Care
(continued)

Medicare pays for <u>acute care</u> services (i.e., hospital care needed to treat a relatively <u>brief episode</u> of illness or accident) but does not provide coverage for <u>chronic care</u> (i.e., personal (physical) care or custodial care needed over a <u>long period</u> for a condition or illness from which an individual may not recover). Medicare, as one of the **hospice care** benefits, will pay for **respite care** or temporary care by a surrogate caregiver to allow the primary caregiver some short-term relief from day-to-day responsibilities. Medicare will not pay for homebound meals ("Meals on Wheels") or **nutritional services** at a senior center.

The major **public sources** for home care coverage consist of Medicare, Medicaid, the Older Americans Act, Social Services and Block Grants. **Non-public sources** (to a limited extent) include privately purchased long-term care insurance, Medicare supplemental insurance, annuities and **out-of-pocket payment**, which may be funded by personal savings, the lifetime use of life insurance policies, or home equity conversions. A wide array of **resources** provide assistance with **information** about home care and related services, including hospital discharge planners, offices for aging, public health and welfare department, nonprofit voluntary agencies (e.g., United Way), **health care agencies (certified or licensed), adult day care centers, senior centers, and churches and synagogues**. In many cases a combination of some of these sources is needed to ensure safety and quality of life at home.

This introductory chapter addresses the following concerns:

- **WHAT DOES THE PATIENT NEED?** (see I below)

- **WHAT TYPES OF HOME CARE ARE AVAILABLE?** (see II below)

- **WHAT IS INVOLVED IN OBTAINING A REPUTABLE HOME CARE AGENCY?** (see III below)

- **WHAT IS INVOLVED IN DIRECT CONTRACTING?** (see IV below)

- **WHAT CARE IS OFFERED BY COMMUNITY AGENCIES?** (see V below)

- **ARE NUTRITION SERVICES AVAILABLE IN THE HOME?** (see VI below)

Chapter 1   **Introduction to Home Care**
(continued)

- **WHERE CAN ONE FIND INFORMATION ON QUALIFIED NURSES, HOME HEALTH CARE AIDES AND HOME CARE WORKERS OR AGENCIES?** (see VII below)

Chapter 1 — Types of Home Care

I. WHAT TYPE OF HOME CARE MAY AN OLDER PERSON NEED? WHAT IS THE COST OF CARE?

A. General

<u>As a general rule, the following questions will determine what types of services and care will be available to the patient, how to apply for the services, how many hours of home care will be needed, how long this care will be available, and how the services will be reimbursed or paid</u>:

- What is the nature of the patient's frailty or illness, and how does it affect the patient's ability to function physically or mentally?
- Does the patient need medically oriented care or non-medical custodial care?
- Will home care be needed on a long-term or short-term basis?
- Has the patient's doctor ordered home care?
- Is the patient eligible for Medicare or Medicaid?
- Does the patient have a private long-term care insurance policy?
- Is the patient able to pay privately for the care that is needed?
- Is the patient capable of directing the home care worker?
- Are family members available who can be called in an emergency?
- Does the home need to be modified to allow for home care equipment?

B. Who Can Help Determine What Care the Patient Needs?

<u>An assessment by a nurse from a **home care agency** can determine exactly what home care assistance the patient needs</u>. A Federal, uniform assessment form has been developed that is used by home health agencies for that purpose.

C. What Is the Average Cost of Home Care?

This question is not easily answered since the cost of home care depends on a variety of factors, including:

Chapter 1   **Types of Home Care**
                                                                                                                                                                               (continued)

- The amount of home care that is needed (this can range from two (2) to twenty-four (24) hours per day);

- How often the home care worker is needed (one day a week or seven days per week);

- What type of home care worker is needed (a trained nurse or therapist, a home health aide, or a personal care aide or housekeeper);

- The degree of the patient's impairment (can the patient be left alone, does the patient need constant attention, how much is the patient able to do herself?); and

- In what part of the country the patient is located.

Home care costs can range from one to several thousand dollars per month. This is one of the reasons why home care is not always less expensive then nursing home care.

Most home care patients need to use a combination of private pay sources, care provided by family and friends, and public benefits.

D.   **Can Family Members Be Paid for the Care They Give the Patient?**

Not most of the time.

The care that is provided by family members and friends, often referred to as "informal care," is not covered by Medicare, Medicaid, or private insurance. Over eighty (80) percent of all care in the home is provided, at no cost to the patient, by such informal caregivers. Many of them supplement the care they give with services obtained from community-based agencies.

In some states, family members can be paid by Medicaid to provide home care.

Chapter 1

Types of Home Care
(continued)

II. WHAT TYPES OF HOME CARE ARE AVAILABLE?

The term "home care" covers many different services that may or may not be paid out of public benefit programs (e.g., Medicare or Medicaid), private insurance, or state programs. <u>Home care consists of medically oriented home care and non-medical home care</u>. Both can be supplemented by other in-home services consisting of nutrition assistance, reassurance programs, day care, socialization, and many other types of community-based services. <u>Differences in the types of required home care will determine how the care will be covered by Medicare or Medicaid and through what type of agency</u>.

A. What Is Medically Oriented Home Care?

Medically oriented home care, usually referred to as "**home health care**," is often needed following an acute medical episode (for example, a heart attack) and is provided under doctor's orders, according to a doctor's plan of care. Home health care is "skilled care" that includes the following:

- <u>Part-time</u> skilled nursing care;
- Physical and occupational therapy and speech language pathology; or
- Hospice care for the terminally ill.

<u>The primary sources of public funding for medically oriented home care are Medicare and Medicaid</u>. Most older Americans are entitled to Medicare, a program that is basically identical in all states; some low-income older Americans may also be eligible for Medicaid, a Federal program that has state and local variations.

B. Is Private Duty Nursing Considered Medically Oriented Care?

Yes.

Recipients of private duty nursing at home are usually persons who would otherwise require hospital care. Although, <u>private duty nursing is not covered by Medicare</u>, it may be funded either under the Medicaid private duty nursing option or through Medicaid waiver programs operated by some states. <u>Private duty nursing must generally be paid out of the patient's personal resources</u>.

Chapter 1   **Types of Home Care**
(continued)

C. What Services Do Home Health Aides Perform?

To qualify as a home health aide, an individual must complete a training program. Such individual under the supervision of skilled medical personnel may perform some medically oriented services, and in addition non-medically oriented services. Home health aide services are delivered under a physician's plan of care and are supervised by a nurse; they include:

- Bandage and dressing changes;
- Help with administering medications (ordered by the doctor);
- Training the patient in self-help skills;
- Help that is supportive of skilled nursing or therapy;
- Routine care of prosthetic devices; and
- The performance of some personal care services.

<u>Home health aide care is reimbursed through Medicare only if it is ordered by the patient's physician in conjunction with skilled services and through Medicaid.</u>

D. What Is Non-medical Home Care?

<u>Non-medical</u> home care consists of home care services that require less training and skills than medical home health care and are performed by personal care aides (called **attendants** or **home care workers**). These services are often referred to as **custodial care** and consist of:

- **Personal care services** including help with bathing, dressing, eating, toileting, transferring (from chair to walker and from bed to wheelchair) turning and positioning; and
- **Homemaker/housekeeping services** including light housework, preparing meals, shopping, laundry and cleaning, and management of money.

<u>Reimbursement for unskilled custodial care is generally not covered by Medicare</u>, except when it is needed in conjunction with medically skilled services such as skilled nursing or skilled therapy. <u>In some states Medicaid will cover non-medical home care services.</u>

Chapter 1   **Types of Home Care**
(continued)

E. **How Does One Obtain a Home Care Worker Privately?**

There are two main approaches to finding a home care worker who will be paid privately, each of which has advantages and disadvantages. In general, patients may be able to obtain care through a home care agency (which can be referred by a hospital discharge planner or an Office for the Aging or a community-based program) or directly by hiring a nurse, home health care aide or home care worker without the assistance of an agency, ideally through word-of-mouth or other recommendation.

F. **How Does One Select an Agency or Home Care Worker?**

The answer to this question depends on the circumstances of the patient. For instance, if the patient is in a hospital or rehabilitation facility, the **facility discharge planner** will develop a discharge plan and will refer the patient to the appropriate home care agency. If the patient is at home and primarily needs custodial care, then the patient may have to obtain home care privately, without the assistance of a discharge planner.

G. **Can a Home Care Worker Be Converted from Private Pay to Coverage under Medicare or Medicaid?**

Yes.

Converting a worker who has been paid privately to Medicare or Medicaid coverage when the home care needs (or the financial situation) of the patient have changed may be possible, but there is no guarantee. Converting the status of the worker from private contracting to employment through an agency depends on whether:

- The worker has the needed training and skills to meet the requirements of the certified home care agency as a vendor of Medicare or Medicaid-covered services;
- The agency is willing to employ the worker; and
- The worker is willing to accept the pay scale of the agency.

H. **What Is a Personal Emergency Response System?**

A personal emergency response system consists of an electronic beeper system, worn by the patient, which is connected to the patient's telephone. A central monitoring station can be activated by the patient, simply by pushing a button on the beeper. This will enable the patient to request help from the central station, even when the patient is unable to use the telephone. If the central station has not heard from the patient after a certain period of time, it will contact the patient to ensure that all is well.

III. WHAT IS INVOLVED IN OBTAINING CARE THROUGH A HOME CARE AGENCY?

Obtaining home care from a home care agency (see Chapter 2, sections I and II) offers the following advantages and disadvantages:

The <u>advantages</u> of obtaining home care through an agency are:

- The home care agency, not the care recipient, is the employer and undertakes the responsibilities of employment, paying taxes, and carrying insurance.

- The agency will arrange for replacement of workers who are ill, unreliable or deemed unsatisfactory.

- The home care patient may choose from among several agencies.

- The home care agency will determine whether the care will be reimbursable through Medicare or Medicaid and submit claims to these sources if the agency is a certified home health agency.

- The services of a **certified home health agency** are monitored for quality control under the Medicare and Medicaid conditions of participation through periodic inspections.

- The services provided by **licensed home care agencies** that do not provide Medicare or Medicaid-covered services are monitored through state licensing regulations.

- A home care agency that is not certified by Medicare or Medicaid, or licensed by a state, may be less expensive than a certified or licensed agency, but the quality of the services may not be as good.

The <u>disadvantages</u> of obtaining home care from a home care agency include:

- It may be difficult to choose from a variety of home care agencies and their reimbursement mechanisms at a time when the patient and informal caregiver(s) may experience stress.

Chapter 1   **Obtaining Care Through a Home Care Agency**
                                                                                                                           (continued)

- Some agencies that are neither licensed nor Medicare/Medicaid-certified are strictly employment agencies that do not train or supervise the home care workers.

Chapter 1   **Direct Contracting**

IV. WHAT IS INVOLVED IN DIRECT CONTRACTING?

The direct payment/contracting approach to home care (as distinct from use of a home care agency) means that the patient or an informal caregiver hires the nurse, home health care aide, or home care worker and contracts directly with the person. Simply put, the patient (or the family) is the employer and is in charge.

The <u>advantages</u> of direct contracting are:

- The ability to select the person best suited to care for the patient (compatibility of personality may be as important as experience or technical skills); and

- The elimination of the middleman, thereby reducing the cost.

The <u>disadvantages</u> of direct contracting are:

- Having the responsibility for hiring and monitoring the nurse, home health care aide, or home care worker and coordinating the care services and related tasks;

- Paying Federal and state unemployment taxes, worker's compensation or disability taxes, and Social Security (FICA) taxes; and

- Obtaining a substitute if the primary nurse, home health care aide or worker is unable to come to work for personal reasons.

Long-term Care at Home Consumer Guide

V. WHAT CARE IS OFFERED BY COMMUNITY AGENCIES?

The in-home care offered by community-based agencies (see Chapter 2, section III) consists of support services that are frequently needed to complement other home care services. They may include:

- Adult social day care;
- Advocacy assistance;
- Transportation;
- Home maintenance tasks;
- Housing improvement;
- Personal emergency response system;
- Telephone reassurance for the patient; and
- Respite care for stressed family members.

The sources of Federal public funding are: <u>Social Services Block Grants, the Older Americans Act, and various Medicaid waiver programs</u>. In addition to Federal programs, many states offer some benefits to augment the services provided in the community.

Chapter 1 — Availability of Nutrition Services

VI. ARE NUTRITION SERVICES AVAILABLE IN THE HOME?

Yes.

A variety of programs provide nutritional assistance to older persons. Nutrition services consist of meals provided to the elderly at home or at **senior centers** (see Chapter 2, section V(C)).

- Home-delivered meals consist of hot, nutritious meals, delivered once and sometimes twice a day, five days a week to persons who are unable to cook for themselves.

- Congregate meals are usually served in senior centers or adult day care programs.

Most nutrition programs are funded through the Federal Older Americans Act and are administered by local Offices for the Aging. There may be a sliding fee (or no fee), determined by the individual's ability to pay.

Food stamps may be available to **homebound** Americans who are eligible for them because they meet the program's financial eligibility requirements. Food stamps consist of debit cards with pre-loaded amounts which can be used to purchase food in most supermarkets.

Chapter 1   Information and Referral Services

VII. WHERE CAN ONE OBTAIN INFORMATION ON QUALIFIED NURSES, HOME HEALTH CARE AIDES, OR HOME CARE WORKERS OR AGENCIES?

In each state and locality, <u>there are sources that provide information about home care and related services</u>. <u>Local Offices for the Aging</u> are often a good source to obtain information about the services available in each locality. Other sources for information or referral include <u>home health agencies, public health and welfare departments, nonprofit voluntary agencies (such as United Way), adult day care centers, senior centers, churches and synagogues</u>. The National Eldercare Locator, which can be reached at (800) 677-1116, provides contact information on the local office for the aging or a community-based family services organization in localities across the country.

Many people who require or desire to pay privately for home care – whether they do so through direct contracting or through a home health agency – <u>will find it helpful to utilize the services of a **geriatric care manager**</u> to obtain information about home care required and then to obtain, screen, monitor and coordinate all of the care services. **Geriatric care managers** are often needed when the patient lives far from family members or friends, who are therefore less capable of monitoring the care and ensuring that the patient's needs are met. **Geriatric care managers** are located in all states, and many are members of the National Association of Professional Geriatric Care Managers, which can be contacted at (520) 881-8008.

CHAPTER 2

WHERE TO OBTAIN HOME CARE

Introduction

Ill or disabled persons who need home care on a short-term or long-term basis face a confusing and complex mosaic of services. Whether they need home care following an acute illness, or because of general physical or mental frailty, obtaining information about services or gaining access to them can be an exhausting experience. The resources available in most communities are quite fragmented. Some agencies offer direct care (medically oriented and/or custodial services), others provide only unskilled care, while some may offer just information referral and advocacy assistance.

This chapter will describe some of the key sources that either offer nurses, home health care agencies, home health aides, home care (personal care) workers or other home care services, or provide information referral, and advocacy assistance. These sources include:

- **CERTIFIED HOME HEALTH AGENCIES** (see section I below);

- **LICENSED HOME CARE AGENCIES** (see section II below);

- **COMMUNITY-BASED AGENCIES** (see section III below);

- **ADULT DAY CARE PROGRAMS** (see section IV below); and

- **AREA AGENCIES ON AGING** (see section V below).

Chapter 2   **Certified Home Health Care Agencies**

I. WHAT ARE CERTIFIED HOME HEALTH CARE AGENCIES?

<u>Many different types of agencies offer home care services</u>. Which agency is the best one for a particular patient depends on the type of care that is needed (medical, non-medical, housekeeping, nutrition assistance, day care) and whether the care is likely to be covered by Medicare, Medicaid, state or local programs, private insurance, or private pay.

Medically oriented services are primarily provided by two types of agencies: <u>certified home health agencies</u>, and <u>licensed home care agencies</u> (see section II).

A **certified home health agency** is a public or private organization that specializes in providing skilled nursing services, skilled therapy services (such as physical and occupational therapy, and speech pathology services), and home health aide services. **Patients who seek Medicare or, in most cases, Medicaid coverage for medically oriented home care must receive these services from a certified home health agency.**

A. What Does "Certified" Mean?

Medicare regulates certified home health agencies in order to protect the interest of Medicare enrollees by imposing so-called **Medicare Conditions of Participation**. These conditions are of importance to agency personnel, who must conform to them, and also to the patients, their families, home care case managers, and advocates who must be aware of the full scope of the obligations of the home care provider as well as the rights and obligations of the patients.

B. What Are Medicare Conditions of Participation?

Conditions of participation for home health agencies require them to:

- Give patients written notice of their rights either before the care relationship begins, or during the initial evaluation visit prior to on the onset of the treatment;

- Maintain the patient's medical records in a confidential manner;

- Advise patients in advance of the cost of care, the portion payable by Medicare and Medicaid, the individual's own payment responsibility, and any changes in charges or payment allocation;

- Abide by all relevant state and Federal laws and regulations;

Chapter 2   **Certified Home Health Care Agencies**
                                                                                                  (continued)

- Disclose the names and addresses of everyone with an ownership or control interest in the agency or who serve as an officer, director, agent, or managing employee of the agency;

- Uphold the rights of patients who are adjudged incompetent by allowing court-appointed guardians or family members to make treatment decisions on their behalf; and

- Inform patients of the right to make a living will or appoint a health care agent (proxy) or both and to include these documents in the patient's medical record. A health care provider may not require patients to have a living will or a health care proxy before it delivers services.

C.   **What Services Are Provided by a Certified Home Health Agency?**

Persons requiring home care and seeking Medicare or Medicaid coverage may obtain the following services from a certified home health agency:

- Skilled nursing services;
- Skilled physical, speech language pathology, and occupational therapy;
- Home health aide services, under supervision of a nurse;
- Medical supplies and equipment;
- Nutritional counseling; and
- Social work services.

D.   **Are Certified Home Health Agency Employees Trained and Supervised?**

Yes. All employees who provide hands-on care must either be licensed health care professionals (registered nurse, licensed practical nurse, licensed therapist) or other competent personnel who have completed a program of training. All home health aides must be trained in recognizing and reporting changes in the patient's condition; emergency procedures; techniques for hygiene; transfers; feeding; and toileting. Home health aides are closely supervised, subject to periodic evaluations, and selected on the basis of such factors as a sympathetic attitude toward the care of the sick, ability to read, write and carry out directions, and maturity and ability to deal effectively with the demands of the job.

E. Are Patients Screened Prior to Obtaining Care?

Yes. Since certified home health agencies offer services that are covered by Medicare or Medicaid, the agencies are also "gate keepers." This means that the home care agencies must determine that services are appropriate for each individual patient, in accordance with the doctor's plan of care, and whether or not the services are likely to be covered by Medicare or Medicaid. Patients may obtain services from the certified home health agency that are not covered by Medicare or Medicaid, as long as they are prepared to pay for the services out of their own resources.

F. What Are the Rights of Certified Home Health Agency Patients?

The rights of the patients who receive home care from a certified home health agency include the right to:

- Expect that the patient's privacy will be respected;
- Voice grievances about quality of care and have a grievance investigated by the agency without reprisals (if the state has a home health hotline for questions and complaints, the patient must be informed of its telephone number and hours of operation);
- Participate in treatment planning and be informed of any change in the plan of care;
- Appeal a denial by Medicare of home care services (see Chapter 3, section V);
- Be informed of the right to make a living will or other advance directive. If the patient has done so, or chooses to do so, the existence and content of the advance directive must be made part of the patient's medical record. However, no health care provider can condition provision of its services on a person either signing or refraining from signing an advance directive.
- Expect that medical records of the patient be kept confidential; and

Chapter 2   **Certified Home Health Care Agencies**
(continued)

- Be advised in advance of the cost of care; the portion payable by Medicare and Medicaid; the individual's own payment responsibility; and any changes in charges or payment allocation.

II. WHAT ARE LICENSED HOME CARE AGENCIES AND THEIR SERVICES?

<u>Some patients who need medically oriented home care may not qualify for Medicare or Medicaid coverage; others may qualify but may choose to obtain nurses, home health aides, or other personnel from licensed home care agencies in order to have greater control over the selection process.</u> Whatever the reasons are for selecting a licensed home care agency, one important factor needs to be highlighted: **licensed home care agencies are not certified by Medicare or Medicaid**, and the services obtained from them are thus not reimbursable by Medicare or Medicaid (however, in some states licensed agencies may contract with a county department of social services to receive Medicaid reimbursement), even though the services may be provided by skilled nurses, therapists, or trained home health aides. Licensed home care providers must meet certain minimum legal standards set by a local, state or government agency.

A. What Services Are Provided by Licensed Home Care Agencies?

Licensed home care agencies provide a variety of home care services to those able to pay for them with their own funds (private payment). The agencies provide these services directly or through contract. The services basically consist of:

- Nursing care;
- Home health aide services; and
- Personal care or home attendant services.

B. Who Uses the Services of Licensed Home Care Agencies?

<u>Even though licensed, the agencies do not provide Medicare and/or Medicaid-covered services. The services are therefore for patients who have the means to pay for home care services out of their own pockets.</u> The advantage of using a licensed home care agency is that the patient and the agency together may develop a service plan that is tailored to the patient's needs. The disadvantages may be that there is less oversight in licensed agencies than in certified agencies, and payment for home care out of one's own resources can be prohibitive for many patients and their families.

C. What Happens When a Patient Depletes His/Her Own Resources?

Once a home care patient has depleted his/her own resources, that patient may be discharged by the licensed home care provider. Or the patient may have become eligible for Medicaid by virtue of having spent down his/her resources and income on medical expenses and thus may be able to obtain home care through Medicaid, depending on whether the state has opted to offer a Medicaid-covered home care program.

If a home care patient begins by paying privately and forms a satisfactory working relationship with a home health care worker from a licensed agency, and then depletes her resources and becomes eligible for Medicaid, it may be possible to keep the same worker after Medicaid eligibility is established if the worker is willing to accept the employment conditions of a Medicaid provider.

III. WHAT ARE COMMUNITY-BASED AGENCIES AND THEIR SERVICES?

In addition to the certified and licensed home care providers, there is a third miscellaneous group of community-based agencies, operating under various auspices, that cover custodial or personal care and housekeeping services. Such agencies and organizations are funded through foundations (e.g., United Way), or other private sources whose function is to provide people with information about where to obtain assistance they may need. Such agencies also may offer supportive services such as: daily money management, recreation, case management, and other services that improve the quality of the patient's life and that may enable the patient to delay nursing home placement.

A. What Services May Be Available from Community Agencies?

Various social welfare agencies and community organizations perform a variety of services that may include:

- Light house cleaning, assistance with personal care and hygiene, and services to assist with heavier chores in the house;
- Free delivery of purchases that have been ordered from drugstores and grocery stores;
- Volunteer services to run local errands, help with small household tasks, or accompany the elderly person to a physician's office;
- Door-to-door transportation services, provided in vans or minibuses which accommodate wheelchairs, walkers and other devices;
- Emergency telephone numbers to dial in times of crises;
- Respite services which provide temporary care for an impaired person in order to relieve family members who provide care to their relative;
- Daily telephone contacts or friendly visiting to reassure patients who live alone by checking in with them and to provide them with a personal contact on a regular basis; and
- A carrier alert program operated by the local post office through which mail carriers watch out for isolated homebound patients.

IV. WHAT ARE ADULT DAY CARE PROGRAMS, THEIR FUNCTIONS, AND FEES?

A. What Are Adult Day Care Programs?

Adult day care centers are proliferating as a community-based source of medical and social services to elderly persons and of respite for family caregivers. There are basically two types of adult day care programs depending upon services rendered:

- <u>Social day care programs</u> emphasize social services, recreation and meals (transportation may or may not be provided). These programs offer little, if any, medical services. Programs that provide no medical services may have to be licensed depending on the participating state.

- <u>Medical day care programs</u>, many of which are affiliated with health care institutions, provide medical, nursing, rehabilitation, and social services, as well as recreation and hot meals on a daily basis to elderly people living in the community. **Transportation** to the program is sometimes provided by the facility. Many day care centers have special programs for Alzheimer's disease patients and others who have lost the ability to be independent. Programs that include medical services are licensed by a state's Department of Health and may be covered by Medicaid or partially covered by Medicare Part B, in addition to the Older Americans Act.

B. Who Are the Main Sources Providing Adult Day Care?

1. <u>States</u>

Several states have statutes providing day care centers. Some illustrations include:

(a) California lets low-income, blind and disabled people use park facilities at off-peak hours; not-for-profit organizations provide bags of food to senior citizens at convenient sites as churches and schools.

(b) Florida provides adult day care centers where basic services are provided to three (3) or more adults, namely, social activities, leisure time activities, self-care training, rest, nutritional services and, where possible, speech and physical therapy and sometimes **transportation** and consumer education.

(c) New York authorizes municipalities to fund and furnish socially adaptive recreation programs for people over age 60 and to receive state aid for these programs.

2. **Corporations and Employees**

Corporations provide for dependent care at a day care center covering parents. This benefit is included as part of a cafeteria plan and funded by salary reduction thereby constituting a non-taxable benefit.

3. **Private Pay**

Adult day care centers created and operated by for-profit entrepreneurs have sprung up throughout the nation,

C. What Are the Different Levels of Adult Day Care?

The National Adult Day Services Association has identified <u>three (3) levels of care provided by adult day care programs</u>. They include core services, enhanced services, and intensive services.

- Participants in need of <u>core services</u> are those whose physical condition is stable, but who require some supervision, supportive services, minimal assistance with activities of daily living, and socialization.

- Individuals needing <u>enhanced services</u> require moderate assistance with none to three (3) activities of daily living, and possibly therapy services at a maintenance level.

- Patients who need <u>intensive services</u> (usually more medically oriented) require maximum assistance, regular monitoring or intervention by a nurse, and possibly therapy services at a rehabilitative or restorative level.

Chapter 2   **Adult Day Care Programs**
                                                                                                                                    (continued)

D.   **Are There Fees for Adult Day Care?**

It depends. <u>The fee of adult day care centers varies</u>. Some centers charge all participants a flat fee, some do not charge any fee, while others may charge a sliding fee depending upon the participant's income.

- In some adult day centers fees may be covered by Medicaid and in part by Medicare.

- Many long-term care insurance policies, where a fixed amount is paid for nursing home and home care, may include adult day care as an additional benefit.

- Some corporations provide dependent care for employee's parents at an adult day care center as part of an employee assistance program. This may be offered free to employees or may be funded by salary reductions, thereby constituting a non-taxable benefit.

E.   **Can Homebound Individuals Receiving Medicare Home Care Coverage Attend Adult Day Care Programs?**

It depends. Attendance at an adult day care center may not cause a Medicare participant to lose coverage as a homebound individual. Absences from home may include attendance at medical adult day centers to receive medical care. The Massachusetts Medicare Advocacy Care Project recommends that the following steps be taken by adult day center providers to better assure continued Medicare coverage:

- Verify the beneficiary's clear medical need to attend the adult day center; and,

- Obtain documentation from the attending physician about the type of medical services that are required of the adult day care provider, and why they are needed.

V. WHAT ARE AREA AGENCIES ON AGING AND THEIR SERVICES?

The Federal government, by enactment of the **Older American's Act**, has created the **Administration on Aging,** a national aging network, that offers a wide range of home and community-based services. Federal funding for these services is distributed to **State Units on Aging**. The state-wide programs are operated at the **local level by Area Agencies on Aging (AAA)**, also called departments of aging or offices for the aging. There are over six-hundred (600) such local agencies in the Untied States; most operate on a county-wide basis. They are nonprofit, public and private organizations, or units of a local government, designated by the state and responsible for a given geographical area to develop and advance plans to advocate on behalf of elderly persons with the greatest economic and social need.

A. Who Is Eligible for Services from an Area Agency on Aging?

All persons <u>age 60 or older</u> are eligible for services. Under the rules of the Older Americans Act, Area Agencies on Aging must give priority to persons with the greatest "economic and social need who are frail and home-bound by reason of illness or disability" or who are isolated. <u>Eligibility for services is determined by the AAA. An applicant does not have to be Medicare or Medicaid-eligible in order to obtain services from an AAA</u>.

B. Does Eligibility for Services Depend on Financial Need?

No. Services provided by AAAs are not subject to means testing, and they are free of charge, although voluntary contributions may be sought. In the case of nutrition services, a fee may be charged according to an individual's ability to pay. Since AAAs also may offer state-specific services that may require a fee or contribution, more specific information should be obtained from the local department for aging.

C. What Services Are Offered by an Area Agency on Aging?

The Older Americans Act is best known as a funding source for the following services:

- **In-home services** may include homemaker and home health aides, personal care services, friendly visiting, telephone reassurance, chore maintenance, respite care for families, adult day care, and minor modification of homes.

- **Nutrition services** may include home-delivered meals, popularly known as "**meals on wheels**," and congregate meals provided at a community or senior center, that are available on a daily basis.

- **In-home respite for a family and adult day care as respite services for a family.**

- **Senior centers** provide the opportunity for social contact, recreation, information and referral, health screening, and education programs. Many offer meals on weekdays, and some have extensive health and social service programs, including adult day care. The centers are an important facility for coordinating and delivering community-based services. In addition to being funded by the Older Americans Act, they may be supported by local governments, philanthropic organizations, participant contributions, and senior volunteers.

- **Long-term care ombudsmen** act as impartial mediators, receiving, investigating and settling complaints from long-term care residents, families or facilities. The state may operate the ombudsman program directly, or it may contract with a local government agency or a private nonprofit organization for this purpose. The ombudsman maintains a staff of volunteers who visit long-term care facilities on a regular basis and work with staff to improve the quality of residents' care.

- **Minor modification of homes** that is necessary to facilitate the ability of older individuals to remain at home and that is not available under other programs.

- **Miscellaneous other services** furnished by AAAs include **transportation**, information and referral, legal assistance, senior employment opportunities, elder abuse protection, and volunteer services for other seniors in the community at large.

CHAPTER 3

ORIGINAL MEDICARE (PARTS A/B)
A FEDERAL SOURCE OF PAYMENT

Introduction

People who need care in the home because of frailty or disability will find that obtaining coverage of home care by Medicare is not a simple matter because of Medicare's qualifying conditions that must be met to establish home care eligibility and its home care service limitations.

Medicare covers only limited home health care.

A. **What Is Medicare?**

Medicare is the **national health insurance program** for people over the age of 65 and for some disabled people under age 65, who must meet certain conditions. Medicare is funded by the Federal government with no state participation (in contrast to Medicaid, the health insurance program for the indigent) and is identical in all states. Medicare's coverage is divided into **Part A – Hospital Insurance**, and **Part B – Supplemental Medical Insurance**. Parts A and B both cover limited home health care if a patient is eligible for and enrolled in Medicare and if the patient meets the required conditions for approval of home health care.

B. **Who Administers the Medicare Program?**

Overall responsibility for the administration of the **Original (Traditional) Medicare Program** rests with the **Secretary of the Department of Health and Human Services** (HHS).

The **Centers for Medicare and Medicaid Services (CMS),** previously known as **Health Care Financing Administration** (HCFA), a division of HHS, directly manages and administers the **Original Medicare** program. Its day-to-day administration of payment of Part A and B bills is operated through private companies under contract with the Secretary of HHS. In the case of **Part A** services, they are called **fiscal intermediaries**, and in the case of **Part B** services (except for **homebound** beneficiaries whose claim administration is through fiscal intermediaries), they are called

| Chapter 3 | Medicare Introduction (continued) |

carriers. The **Medicare Prescription Drug and Improvement Modernization Act** of 2003 (MMA) mandates that the Secretary of HHS replace the fiscal intermediaries and the carriers with **Medical Administrative Contractors.** The full implementation of this program is scheduled for completion in 2011.

Medicare independent review entities, consisting of groups of practicing physicians and other health care experts, participate (as private contractors for HHS) in the administration of the Medicare program. These entities are called **Quality Improvement Organizations** (QIO) (formerly known as **Peer Review Organizations** (PRO)). The QIO's functions consist of the following: (i) responsibility for making determinations regarding the necessity and reasonableness of health care provided by Medicare; (ii) reviewing of **non-coverage notices** issued by hospitals to Medicare beneficiaries changing coverage of their continued stay; (iii) evaluating the efficiency and economy of the health care services provided; (iv) ensuring that such services meet professional and accepted medical quality of care standards; and (v) reviewing the professional activities of prescription drug sponsors pursuant to contracts under **Medicare Part D**. In addition, the QIOs review complaints by beneficiaries relating to the quality of care in settings such as in-patient hospitals, hospital outpatient departments, hospital emergency rooms, **skilled nursing facilities, home health agencies, private fee-for-service** plans, and ambulatory sites. QIOs make **Initial Determinations** in hospital cases, but do not issue payments; they authorize the appropriate contractor to issue payment.

CMS has established new entities called **Qualified Independent Contractors** (QIC) to conduct a second level of administrative reviews (called **Reconsideration(s)**) of Part A claims and denials made by fiscal intermediaries, carriers and QIOs.

C. Do Medicare-eligibles Receive an Identification Card?

Yes. Medicare-eligible persons receive a **Medicare Health Service** card in the mail following an application for Medicare or in certain cases automatically. The card is red, white and blue. It shows the name of the Medicare person, his/her **Medicare claim number** (Social Security number), entitlement to **Hospital Insurance (Part A)** and/or **Supplemental Medical Insurance (Part B)**, and the effective date of each.

If the Medicare eligible should lose or damage the Medicare health insurance card, he/she can order a new card online at

Chapter 3	Medicare Introduction
	(continued)

www.socialsecurity.gov (selecting a number from the "subject" list) or by calling the Social Security Administration at 1-800-772-1213. Persons who are deaf, hard of hearing or have speech impairments can call 1-800-325-0778.

This chapter describes the following aspects of Medicare:

- **ELIGIBILITY REQUIREMENTS FOR MEDICARE PARTS A AND B** (see section I below)

- **ENROLLMENT PROCEDURES FOR MEDICARE PARTS A AND B** (see section II below)

- **REQUIREMENTS (QUALIFYING CONDITIONS) THAT HAVE TO BE MET IN ORDER TO OBTAIN MEDICARE COVERAGE OF HOME HEALTH SERVICES** (see section III below)

- **HOSPICE CARE** (see section IV below)

- **APPEALS** (see section V below)

- **MEDICARE AS A SECONDARY PAYER** (see section VI below)

- **PROGRAM FOR ALL-INCLUSIVE CARE FOR THE ELDERLY** (see section VII below)

- **PHYSICIANS OPTING OUT OF MEDICARE** (see section VIII below)

- **COORDINATION OF COVERAGE BETWEEN MEDICARE AND AN EMPLOYER PLAN** (see section IX below)

- **CONTINUATION OF COVERAGE UNDER INSURANCE PLAN OF PRIOR EMPLOYER (COBRA)** (see section X below)

- **SERVICES IN ADDITION TO OR SUPPLEMENTAL TO HOME CARE** (see section XI below)

Long-term Care at Home Consumer Guide

Chapter 3   Eligibility Requirements

I. WHAT ARE THE ELIGIBILITY REQUIREMENTS FOR MEDICARE?

A. Who Is Eligible for Medicare Part A?

The following categories of persons are eligible for Medicare Part A:

- Persons age 65 and over, entitled to receive either **Social Security** or **Railroad Retirement** benefits. Also eligible are **spouses** or **former spouses** of these persons who qualify for Social Security benefits as dependents and who have attained 65 years of age.

    Note: Persons who elect retirement at age 62 are not eligible for **Medicare** until they turn 65. Persons who elect to postpone **Social Security** retirement benefits and continue working after age 65 can begin receiving **Medicare** benefits at age 65.

    Note: Employers with 20 or more employees must offer employees over age 65 the option of receiving the same private health insurance package that they offer other employees in lieu of, or in addition to, receiving Medicare.

- Persons under age 65 who have received **Social Security** or **Railroad Retirement** disability benefits for twenty-four (24) months. **Eligibility** begins on the twenty-fifth (25th) month. Medicare benefits will continue up to ninety-three (93) months after the individual has stopped receiving **disability benefits** because of successfully completing a nine- (9) month trial work period.

- Transitional group of persons, not eligible for **Social Security** or **Railroad Retirement** benefits, who reached age 65 before 1968 or who became age 65 and had three (3) quarters of coverage for each year between 1967 and 1974.

- Persons under age 65 with **end-stage renal disease** who require **dialysis** or a **kidney transplant** (if fully insured or currently insured or if the wife or **dependent** child of such insured person). Most of these persons are eligible for Medicare benefits after a three- (3) month **waiting period**. The **waiting period** does not apply to **transplant** candidates, provided their

Chapter 3 **Eligibility Requirements**
(continued)

surgery takes place before the third month or to individuals who participate in a self-care training program before the beginning of the third month.

- Persons diagnosed with **amyotrophic lateral sclerosis** who receive either **Social Security** or **Railroad Retirement disability benefits**.

- **Employees of the Federal government from 1983 on, as well as state and local government employees hired after March 1986**. In each case these government employees must have the required work credits (quarters of coverage) under the **Social Security** program and meet several other technical requirements. **Dependents** and **survivors** of these workers are also covered.

- **Voluntary enrollees** who: (a) attained age 65, (b) are not eligible for either **Social Security** or **Railroad Retirement** benefits, (c) are residents of the United States, <u>and</u> (d) are either citizens of the United States or **aliens** lawfully admitted for permanent residence (who have continuously resided in the United States for not less than five years immediately before the month in which **application** for enrollment is made). These individuals may purchase Medicare coverage by payment of a monthly **premium** that CMS determines annually ($423/month in 2008). In order for a **voluntary enrollee** to receive coverage in **Medicare Part A**, he/she must enroll in **Medicare Part B**.

B. Who Is Eligible for Medicare Part B?

Medicare Part B is a voluntary program for eligible individuals who enroll in the program and who pay a **premium**, or by having it deducted from their monthly Social Security check ($96.40/month in 2008). <u>Eligibility for Part B does not depend on Part A eligibility</u>, although all individuals age 65 eligible for Part A are automatically entitled to Part B. **An individual age 65 or over is eligible for enrollment for Part B if he/she is either entitled to hospital insurance under Part A or is a United States resident who is either an American citizen or a permanent resident alien who has resided in the United States for the five (5) years immediately before the month of application for enrollment.**

Chapter 3

Eligibility Requirements
(continued)

C. What Happens When People Cannot Afford Monthly Premiums?

Several categories of Medicare enrollees are known as low-income Medicare beneficiaries. These individuals are entitled to have Medicare premiums and other payments <u>paid by Medicaid</u> if <u>they meet certain income and asset requirements</u>. Starting with the lowest income/resource group, the categories include:

- *Qualified Medicare Beneficiaries.* Payment of deductibles and co-payment costs under Parts A and B, and Medicare premiums under Part B and in some cases under Part A.

- *Specified Low-income Medicare Beneficiaries.* Payment of Medicare premiums under Part B, subject to certain limitations.

- *Qualifying Individuals.* Payment of Medicare Part B premiums.

- *Qualified Disabled and Working Individuals.* Payment of Medicare premiums under Part B only.

D. Can People Have Both Medicare and Medicaid?

Yes. The low-income Medicare enrollees listed in the previous question qualify for Medicaid. When people qualify for both Medicare and Medicaid eligibility, they are known as **dual eligibles**. In those situations Medicare is the primary payer, followed by Medicaid.

E. Can People Have Both Medicare and Employer-Paid Health Insurance?

Yes. Some people have both Medicare and employer-paid health insurance. For Medicare beneficiaries who are still employed, Medicare is the secondary payer. However, for retirees who are no longer working and who have employer-paid health insurance, Medicare will be the primary payer.

Chapter 3   Enrollment Requirements

II. WHAT ARE THE MEDICARE ENROLLMENT REQUIREMENTS AND PROCEDURES?

A. How Does One Enroll in Medicare?

The enrollment process for Medicare Part A is automatic for many people, but some people must file a separate application to enroll in Medicare Parts A and B.

B. Who Is Eligible for Automatic Enrollment?

1. Part A

Enrollment is automatic for most persons age 65 or older who are entitled to and are receiving Social Security or Railroad Retirement benefits. Application by these persons for these benefits is considered to be an application for Medicare **Part A** and **Part B** (unless they indicate they do not want Part B), and automatically triggers the **enrollment** process without the necessity of a separate application.

Enrollment is also **automatic** for a person, irrespective of age, who has been a **disability** patient receiving benefits under the **Social Security Act** or **Railroad Retirement Act** for twenty-four (24) months. Such patient will automatically receive his/her Medicare card for **Part A** and **Part B benefits**.

Should a person be eligible for **Social Security** or **Railroad Retirement** benefits but not be receiving **those** benefits, then eligibility for **Medicare Part A** is not automatic, and he/she must file an **application**.

2. Part B

Persons age 65 or older who are entitled to Social Security or Railroad Retirement benefits and are receiving such benefits are automatically eligible for Medicare Part B. As in the case of **Medicare Part A**, a separate Medicare enrollment for Part B is unnecessary.

Should an individual fail to file an application during the **initial enrollment period**, then he/she will be subject to a **late enrollment**

Chapter 3

Enrollment Requirements (continued)

charge and will not be able to enroll until the next **general enrollment period** (January 1 -- March 31). If a person enrolls for **Part B** benefits during the **general enrollment period**, coverage will not begin until July of that year (see section E below).

As in the case of **Medicare Part A benefits**, a person age 65 or over who is a U.S. citizen or a permanent **resident alien** residing in the United States for at least five (5) years immediately prior to application, can purchase **Medicare Part B** benefits by filing an application and paying monthly **premiums** which CMS fixes annually.

C. Who Has to Apply Separately to Enroll?

Should a person be eligible for **Social Security** or **Railroad Retirement** benefits but not be receiving **those** benefits, then eligibility for **Medicare Part A** is not automatic, and he/she must file an **application**. Individuals who are eligible for Social Security or Railroad Retirement benefits but are not receiving those benefits will not be automatically eligible for Medicare Part B benefits and must file an application for Part B benefits. As is the case of Medicare Part A, the application for Part B coverage should be filed during the initial enrollment period to maximize the entitlement benefits.

The filing of an application also relates to persons age 65 or older who are entitled to retirement benefits but have elected to postpone retirement and continue working after age 65. These persons are eligible for Medicare, but to obtain Medicare benefits, they must file an application for enrollment during one of the three enrollment periods.

People who are not eligible for Social Security or Railroad Retirement benefits because they never paid the necessary taxes (or did not pay into the systems for the required period of time) may purchase Medicare Part A or B by paying monthly premiums for both (see section I.A about voluntary enrollees).

D. When Are the Enrollment Periods?

There are basically three different enrollment periods:

- ***Initial enrollment period.*** This is a period of seven (7) months. It begins with the third month prior to the month when the prospective enrollee reaches age 65 and continues

Chapter 3   **Enrollment Requirements**
                                                                       (continued)

for three (3) months after the month of his/her 65th birthday. **If an individual does not file during the initial enrollment period, then he/she can file during the general enrollment period.**

Enrollment during the first three (3) months of the initial enrollment period will result in coverage the first day of the month the individual attains age 65. Enrollment after the first three (3) months will cause a delay in coverage. Enrollment in the month when the beneficiary reaches age 65 will result in coverage on the first day of the second month after the applicant enrolls. If the applicant enrolls during the last three (3) months of the **initial enrollment period**, there may be a delay in coverage of one (1) to three (3) months.

Should a voluntary enrollee file an application after the initial enrollment period, a Part A and Part B penalty surcharge will be imposed. Should other Medicare-eligible persons file an **application** after the **initial enrollment period**, no Part A **penalty** will be imposed. However, such individuals, except those specified in **special enrollment period** (see below), will be subject to a Part B penalty **surcharge**.

- *Annual general enrollment period.* This is held during the period January 1 through March 31 of each year. Coverage begins on July 1 after the application is filed.

- *Special enrollment period.* This period relates to working individuals age 65 or over who are covered by an **employer group health plan** whether it be his/her own or that of a **spouse**. <u>These persons have the option to enroll in Medicare after age 65</u>. The enrollment period begins on the first day of the month in which the person is no longer enrolled in an **employer group plan** and ends seven (7) months later. Enrollment will not result in any **penalty** payment of **late enrollment** charges.

E. What Happens If an Application Is Not Filed on Time?

Should an individual fail to file an application during the initial enrollment period (or the special enrollment period for employed individuals), then <u>he or she will be subject to a penalty charge on the Part B premium</u> and will not be able to enroll until the next general enrollment period (January 1 -- March 31). If a person enrolls for Part B benefits during the general enrollment period, coverage will not begin until July of that year.

Chapter 3 — Home Health Care Requirements

III. WHAT ARE THE REQUIREMENTS FOR MEDICARE-COVERED HOME HEALTH CARE?[*]

A. How Does One Qualify for Medicare-covered Home Health Care?

When a patient applies for limited Medicare-covered home health care, a certified home health agency will assess the patient and determine whether or not the patient meets **five Medicare Qualifying Conditions** and whether the patient needs **Qualifying Skilled Services**. <u>The home health qualifying conditions must be met, and the need for skilled services must be established in order to obtain Medicare-covered home health care.</u>

If a patient does not meet the qualifying conditions or if he/she does not need either intermittent skilled nursing care or skilled therapy, then he/she will not be able to obtain Medicare coverage for those needs.

Once a patient has been found to be eligible for home health coverage under Medicare because the patient meets the Qualifying Conditions and has a need for Qualifying Skilled Services, then the patient is also entitled to **Dependent Services**.

B. What Are the Five Medicare Qualifying Conditions?

The Medicare Qualifying (eligibility) Conditions include:

- The needed home care must be **reasonable and necessary**; (see 1 below)

- The patient must be **homebound**; (see 2 below)

- The patient must obtain a **plan of care** from the physician, prescribing the needed services; (see 3 below)

- The patient must need **Qualifying Skilled Services, "intermittent" skilled nursing care, or therapy**; (see 4 below)

- The patient must obtain the services from a **Medicare-certified home health agency**. (see 5 below)

---

[*] Medicare Part B will help pay for certain services and supplies in addition to home health care (see Appendices A-F, and chapter XI below).

Long-term Care at Home Consumer Guide   © 2009 Walter Feldesman

Chapter 3

Home Health Care Requirements
(continued)

1. **<u>What is meant by reasonable and necessary?</u>**

   In order to be considered reasonable and necessary, the services must be consistent with the nature **and** severity of the patient's illness or injury, his or her particular medical needs, and accepted standards of medical and nursing care. This determination must be based solely upon the patient's unique condition, without regard to whether the illness or injury is acute, chronic, terminal, or expected to last a long time.

   Therapy services must be provided with the expectation, based upon a physician's assessment of the patient's potential, that his/her condition will improve materially in a reasonable and generally predictable length of time or that the services are necessary for the establishment of a safe maintenance program.

2. **<u>What is meant by homebound?</u>**

   Homebound is the inability to leave home without assistance because of an illness or injury. The patient must be confined to the home but not necessarily bedridden. The patient can leave the home if absences are infrequent and for short durations, or are for necessary medical treatment.

3. **<u>What is meant by a physician's plan of care?</u>**

   In order to be covered by Medicare, all home care services must be provided under a physician's plan of care. The plan does not require a narrative description of the services ordered but must specify the medical treatments to be furnished, who will furnish them, and the frequency they will be furnished. The physician's plan of care is also needed for therapy, and the doctor may consult with a therapist prior to writing the plan. It must be signed and dated by the physician, and while verbal orders are permissible, they must be countersigned by the physician in a timely fashion and dated by the physician before the home health agency bills for the care. Finally, the physician must review the plan of care at least once every sixty-two (62) days. Each review must contain the signature of the physician and the date of review.

Long-term Care at Home Consumer Guide

Chapter 3   Home Health Care Requirements
(continued)

4. <u>**What are the qualifying skilled services?**</u>

The patient's physician must determine whether the patient needs skilled services. In order for a service to be considered skilled, the care that is provided must be medically oriented and must be performed by a registered nurse, licensed practical nurse, or licensed therapist. If a service can be safely and effectively performed by the average non-medical person, then it is <u>not</u> a skilled service.

(a) **Skilled nursing** must be performed by a registered nurse or licensed practical (vocational) nurse. Skilled nursing excludes any service that could be safely and effectively performed or self-administered by the average non-medical person without the direct intervention of a licensed nurse. It makes no difference if a patient's condition is acute, chronic or terminal. Examples of what constitutes skilled nursing care are:

- observation and assessment of a patient's condition;

- performance of skilled procedures such as tube feeding, catheter care, wound care, kidney dialysis, colostomy care, changing specific dressings, and injections;

- management and evaluation of the patient's care plan, as established by the patient's doctor;

- supervision of non-skilled personnel; and

- teaching or training family members to provide care that is needed and that can be performed by them.

(a-1) **"Intermittent" Defined**

In order for a nursing service to be considered "intermittent," the care must be needed less than daily, or, if daily, less than eight (8) hours each day for a relatively short period of time twenty-one (21) days or less) with extensions permitted in exceptional circumstances when the need for additional care is finite and predictable.

Chapter 3   **Home Health Care Requirements**
(continued)

(b) **Skilled therapy** includes physical therapy and speech-language pathology. Occupational therapy is counted as a Qualifying Skilled Service only if the therapist is licensed and if it is part of a care plan which also includes intermittent skilled nursing, physical therapy, or speech-language pathology services. Medicare has imposed annual limits on the amount of skilled therapy services covered on an outpatient basis. <u>The annual limit on the allowed amount of outpatient physical therapy and speech pathology combined is $1,810 (2008); the limit for occupational therapy is $1,810 (2008)</u>. The limits apply to outpatient Part B therapy services from all settings including outpatient hospital services and hospital emergency rooms.

Therapy may be provided in the patient's home or outside of the home (see Appendix A). The therapy must relate directly and specifically to a treatment regimen (established by the physician, after any needed consultation with the qualified therapist) that is designed to treat the beneficiary's illness or injury. Services related to activities for the general physical welfare of beneficiaries (for example, exercises to promote overall fitness, unrelated to the patient's illness) are not considered skilled therapy services for Medicare purposes.

5. **What is meant by "certified" home health agency?**

In order to be covered by Medicare, <u>all services must be supplied by a home health care agency that is "certified" by Medicare</u>.

C. **What Are the Dependent Services?**

If any of the skilled services is provided, then five <u>Dependent Services</u> may be available, including the following:

- **"Part-time or intermittent" home health aides** (see 1 below). Medicare will cover twenty-eight <u>(28) to thirty-five (35) hours per week of a combination of nursing and home health aide services</u>. However, Medicare frequently limits the extent of home health aide services because of the reasonable and necessary standard. This means that although use of home health aides theoretically is available for extended periods, <u>Medicare frequently limits the visits of home</u>

health aides to three (3) or four (4) hours per day for a few days per week (see 1 below).

- **medical social services** if supervised by a physician (see 2 below);

- durable medical equipment (see 3 below);

- **medical supplies** (other than drugs and biologicals) (see 4 below); and

- **services of interns or residents**, if the certified home health agency is affiliated with a hospital that has an approved medical education program (see 5 below).

1. **Home health aides**

    (a) **What is a home health aide?**

    A home health aide is a person who performs semi-skilled tasks under the supervision of a licensed practical nurse. Home health aides must successfully complete an approved training program and receive at least twelve (12) hours of in-service training during each twelve- (12) month period. In order to be covered by Medicare, the services of the home health aide must be ordered by the physician and described in the plan of care.

    (b) **What are the duties of a home health aide?**

    Home health aide services include, but are not limited to:

    - hands-on personal care that is supportive of skilled nursing activities, such as: bathing; dressing; grooming needed to facilitate treatment or prevent deterioration of the patient's health; changing the bed linens of an incontinent patient; skin, foot, and ear care; feeding; assistance with elimination;

transfers and ambulation; and changing the patient's position in bed;

- simple dressing changes that do not require the skills of a licensed nurse;

- assistance with medications that do not require the skills of a licensed nurse to be provided safely and effectively;

- assistance with activities that are directly supportive of skilled therapy services but do not require the skills of a therapist;

- assistance in ambulation or exercise; and

- routine care of prosthetic and/or orthotic devices.

(c) **Does a home health aide provide housekeeping services?**

No. Housekeeping tasks or **homemaker** services, such as cooking meals, dishwashing, doing laundry or shopping, are generally <u>not covered by Medicare</u>.

2. **Medical social services**

Medical social services include the following:

- counseling of the patient that is necessary to resolve social or emotional problems that are expected to be an impediment to the effective treatment of the patient's medical condition or to his or her rate of recovery; and

- family counseling services, ordered by a physician when the primary purpose is the treatment of the beneficiary's condition and not the treatment of a family member's condition.

Medical social services must be furnished by a qualified social worker, or a qualified social worker assistant under the supervision of a social worker, and they must be provided under the direction of a physician and be included in the plan of care prepared by the physician.

3. **Durable medical equipment** (see Appendix D)

    Examples of durable medical equipment include: iron lungs, canes, oxygen tents, hospital beds, wheelchairs, walkers, and seat lift chairs. To be considered durable medical equipment, the equipment must be:

    - re-usable by other patients;
    - needed primarily for a medical purpose;
    - appropriate for use in the patient's home; and
    - necessary and reasonable for the treatment of the patient's illness or injury or to improve the functioning of the patient.

    The patient is required to pay twenty (20) percent of the approved charges as coinsurance payment if the provider accepts assignment. If the provider does not accept assignment, patients are required to pay the coinsurance and any amount above Medicare's approved amount, charged by the provider. Under certain conditions, patients may elect to purchase an item of equipment rather than rent it.

4. **Medical supplies**

    Two types of medical supplies are covered by Medicare on the basis of a home visit:

    - Routine medical supplies are customarily used during the course of most home care visits by home health agency staff and are not designated for a specific patient (for example, swabs, thermometers, and masks); and

Chapter 3   **Home Health Care Requirements**
(continued)

- Non-routine supplies that must be specifically ordered by a physician for use in treating a specific patient (for example, catheters, splints, syringes, and sterile dressings).

Prescription drugs and biologicals are not considered medical supplies and are not covered by Medicare home health care benefits or as part of Medicare outpatient treatment. However, they may be covered as a Medicare hospice benefit.

5. **Services of Interns and Residents**

The services of interns and residents are covered under a physician's plan of care; ordered by the physician who is responsible for the plan; and obtained through a home health agency that is affiliated with or under the common control of the hospital furnishing the medical services of interns and residents in training under an approved hospital teaching program.

The need for such services must be reasonable and necessary for the diagnosis or treatment of a beneficiary's illness or injury, or to improve the functioning of the patient.

Chapter 3   Home Health Care Requirements
                                                                              (continued)

D. What Types of Home Care Services Are Not Covered by Medicare?

Medicare does not cover the following types of home care services:

- Personal (custodial) care, customarily rendered by **a personal care aide**. This is an unskilled service that assists elderly persons with activities commonly called **activities of daily living,** such as bathing and feeding. These services <u>may</u> be covered by Medicare to a limited extent when they are performed by a home health aide, prescribed by the patient's physician, and <u>only if they are incidental to Medicare skilled nursing or therapy services</u>.

- Non-skilled services, such as assistance with instrumental activities of daily living, including preparing meals, shopping, and light housework.

- Community-based services such as homebound meals (meals on wheels) or congregate meals.

- Management and coordination of services, such as case management.

E. Are There Out-of-Pocket Costs When Receiving Medicare Home Care?

That depends. If the patient's needs can be met by the intermittent skilled and dependent care that is available through Medicare, then the patient has no out-of-pocket costs for home care. **Medicare does not require co-payments or deductibles for Medicare-covered home care, except for twenty (20) percent of the allowable cost of durable medical equipment.** However, if the patient's needs are not fully met by the care that is covered by Medicare (for instance, when the patient needs housekeeping services or other non-skilled care), then the home care must be supplemented by other non-Medicare services that will generate additional costs.

In general, patients should expect to have additional costs because, at a minimum, most home care patients require outpatient care that is never reimbursed by Medicare, such as homemaker services, eye glasses or hearing aids, routine foot care, and transportation.

Chapter 3 — Medicare-covered Hospice Care

IV. WHAT IS HOSPICE CARE, AND WHAT DOES MEDICARE COVER?

Hospice services are neither within the category of skilled home health services nor dependent services. They are separate services covered by Part A. They will only be furnished at the election of a Medicare enrollee, instead of standard Medicare benefits. Hospice care must be provided by a **certified hospice program**. It may be provided in the patient's home, but may also be offered in a hospital or a separate hospice facility. Hospice services consist of care covered by Medicare Part A that is specially designed for persons who are terminally ill. Hospice programs emphasize relieving pain and managing symptoms rather than focusing on healing or a cure.

A. Who Is Eligible for Hospice Care?

In order to be eligible for hospice care, **a patient must be terminally ill** and have a life expectancy of six (6) months or less. A terminally ill patient may elect to receive hospice care rather than regular Medicare benefits for the management of his/her terminal illness. By selecting hospice care, the patient agrees to forego any alternative care that has the intention to heal the patient. A hospice patient may revoke the election of hospice care at any time and restore eligibility to regular Medicare benefits.

B. What Are the Qualifying Conditions for Medicare Hospice Care?

In order to obtain Medicare-covered hospice care, the patient must meet the following four conditions:

- The attending physician -- either in the employ of the hospice, or under contract with the hospice as an independent physician or as part of an independent physicians group -- and the medical director of the hospice must establish and periodically review a written plan for hospice care, and certify that the patient is **terminally ill**, with a life expectancy of six (6) months or less.

- The patient must elect to receive care from a hospice instead of standard Medicare medical benefits for the terminal illness. Should a patient revert to standard Medicare benefits he or she will then be required to pay any applicable deductibles and co-payments.

- Care must be provided by a Medicare-certified hospice program.

- The individual must be eligible for Part A benefits.

C. What Services Are Included in Medicare Hospice Care?

If the conditions as outlined above are met, Medicare will pay for the following services:

- nursing services;

- doctors' services;

- drugs, including outpatient drugs for pain relief and symptom management;

- physical, occupational, and speech-language therapy;

- home health aides and **homemaker** services,

- medical social services;

- medical supplies (including drugs and biologicals) and appliances;

- short-term inpatient care including both respite care and procedures necessary for pain control and acute and chronic symptom management;

- training and counseling for the patient and family members; and

- any other item or service which is specified in the plan of care.

Chapter 3   **Medicare-covered Hospice Care**
                                                                                                                                (continued)

      Medicare pays for up to two (2) ninety- (90) day periods of hospice care followed by an unlimited number of sixty- (60) day periods as long as the patient remains terminally ill.

Chapter 3   Appealing Medicare Home Care Denials

V. WHAT IS THE APPEAL PROCESS FOR HOME CARE DENIALS, REDUCTIONS, OR TERMINATION OF SERVICES?

A. What Are the Steps Prior to an Appeal?

In order to appeal a decision, <u>a patient must first apply for home health care by contacting a certified home health agency</u> (CHHA) that has a contractual obligation to assess the patient's needs and eligibility for Medicare coverage, to provide the services, and submit the patient's claim to the Medicare fiscal intermediary (FI).

When the certified home health agency determines that a patient's claim for Medicare coverage is likely to be authorized by Medicare, no advance notice is required, and the agency will provide home care and then submit the patient's claim for coverage to the FI. After the home health agency sends the claim to the Medicare intermediary, Medicare will forward to the Medicare beneficiary a **Medicare summary notice** (MSN) for Part A and/or Part B services. The MSN will inform beneficiary of the FI's determination on the claim. The MSN is not a bill. It represents the initial Medicare Determination and lists the services received by the beneficiary and the amount he/she may be billed for them. The MSN will inform the beneficiary of the determination by the FI on the claim and his/her right to appeal the determination.

If the FI determines not to cover the claim submitted by the home care agency, then the patient has a right to appeal this decision within one-hundred twenty (120) days of the date the beneficiary received the MSN.

When the CHHA determines at the outset that a patient's claim for Medicare coverage is not likely, that a service provided in the course of treatment be reduced, or that a specific service(s) among several provided during treatment be terminated, it must give the patient a notice called **Home Health Advance Beneficiary Notice**. If the patient insists on obtaining the care he or she feels is needed, the home care agency will provide home care services and bill the patient directly, and the patient will be responsible for home care payment (see B below).

When the CHHA determines to terminate services completely, it must give the beneficiary advance notice to this effect. This notice informs the beneficiary when Medicare coverage ends and includes the beneficiary's **appeal** rights (see B below).

Chapter 3   **Appealing Medicare Home Care Denials or Reductions**
(continued)

B. Can a Patient Appeal an Advance Notice to the Beneficiary from the Home Care Agency?

No. The home care agency's notice is not the same as a Medicare determination from a fiscal intermediary and cannot be appealed to the Medicare system. The notice does not form the basis of an appeal. The beneficiary must obtain a formal Medicare determination. The Medicare Summary Notice constitutes the Initial Determination and briefly explains what Medicare will pay on a claim.

The home health agency has certain obligations that patients should be aware of:

- Home health agencies must provide the home care services that have been requested by the patient (even when the agency does not believe Medicare will cover them) as long as the patient agrees to pay privately.

- If services have started, the patient may demand that the agency submit the bill to the Medicare fiscal intermediary. (This is referred to as **demand billing.**) Once the home care agency has submitted the bill to the fiscal intermediary, the fiscal intermediary, acting for Medicare, will decide whether or not to pay for the services. If the intermediary decides to deny the claim, the patient has the right to appeal the Medicare decision.

Chapter 3   **Appealing Medicare Home Care Denials or Reductions (continued)**

C. What Is the Medicare Part A and Part B Appeals Process of Home Health Claims?

1. General

If a fiscal intermediary (FI) denies a claim (**initial determination**), it must notify the home health agency, and the beneficiary of the denial and offer the beneficiary the opportunity to appeal its decision. The determination can be appealed.

There is a uniform process for handling Part A and Part B claims, including a new level of appeal for appeal of claims before a newly established entity, the **Qualified Independent Contractor (QIC)**. The appeal process embraces the following:

2. Standard Appeal Process

These are the levels of appeal:

- Initial Determinations by the FI. When the FI makes a determination (called "Initial Determination") with respect to a claim, the beneficiary may appeal the determination, and seek re-determination from the FI.

- Re-determination by the FI. **This is the first level of appeal**. The FI will make a re-determination of its initial determination.

- Reconsideration by the QIC. If the FI upholds its re-determination, **this is the second level of appeal by the beneficiary**. The QIC, a new review entity, will reconsider the re-determination of the FI.

- Hearing before the Administrative Law Judge (ALJ). If the QIC upholds the re-determination decision of the FI, **this is the third level of appeal by the beneficiary**. The ALJ will review the reconsideration decision of the QIC.

- Review by Departmental Appeals Board (DAB). If the ALJ upholds the reconsideration decision by the QIC, this is the **fourth level of appeal by the beneficiary**. The DAB will review the ALJ decision.

- Federal District Court. If the DAB upholds the ALJ decision, **this is the final level of appeal**.

Chapter 3 — Appealing Medicare Home Care Denials or Reductions (continued)

The following chart illustrates the five levels in the standard appeal process, the amount in controversy (AIC) to qualify for an appeal, the number of days to file an appeal, and the time limit for a decision.

Five Levels of the Standard Appeal Process	
Initial Determination by FI • The required Amount in Controversy (AIC) – $0 • The number of days to file an appeal for Re-determination by the FI of the Initial Determination – 120 days	**Third Level of Appeal – ALJ Hearing** • The required AIC - $120 • The time limit for ALJ decision – 90 days • The number of days to file for review by DAB – 60 days
First Level of Appeal – Re-determination by FI • The required AIC – $0 • Time limit for a **Re-determination** – 180 days • The number of days to file for a **Reconsideration** by the QIC – 60 days	**Fourth Level of Appeal – DAB Review** • The required AIC – $0 • The time limit for DAB decision – None • The number of days to file appeal to the federal District Court – 60 days
Second Level of Appeal – Reconsideration by the QIC • The required AIC – $0 • The time limit for a **Reconsideration** by the AIC – 60 days • The number of days to file appeal for a hearing to ALJ – 60 days	**Final Appeal – Federal District Court** • The required AIC – $1,180 • The time limit for decision – None

Long-term Care at Home Consumer Guide

3. **Expedited Appeal Process for Termination of Services by Home Health Agency (HHA)**

(a) **Provider's Advance Notice of Termination.**

Before any complete termination of services, the HHA must deliver a written notice (called "**Notice of Medicare Provider Non-coverage**") informing the beneficiary of the HHA's decision to **terminate services.** This notice requirement applies only to complete termination of services but does not apply to any reduction of services or termination of a specific service during a course of treatment. The HHA must give such notice to the beneficiary no later than two (2) days before the proposed end of the services and must provide a description of the beneficiary's right to obtain an Expedited Determination by the Quality Improvement Organization (QIO) of whether the HHA's decision was correct, and how to request an Expedited Determination and Expedited Reconsideration. **Beneficiaries may seek such expedited determinations.** The steps of such process are as follows:

(b) **Expedited Determination.**

- A Request by Beneficiary. A beneficiary, who wishes to exercise the right to an Expedited Determination, must submit a request for such determination to the **QIO** by no later than the noon of the calendar day following receipt of the HHA's notice.

- Continuing Coverage. The coverage of the HHA's services will continue until the date and time designated in the notice.

- Notice by QIO. On the day that the **QIO** receives a request for Expedited Determination, it must notify the HHA that a request for an Expedited Determination has been made.

    The HHA must send a second notice, called a Detailed Explanation of Non-Coverage, to the beneficiary by the close of business of the QIO's notification, setting forth why the services are either no longer necessary or no longer covered.

Chapter 3   **Expedited Appeal Process**

- QIO's Determination. Not later than seventy-two (72) hours after receipt of the beneficiary's request for an **Expedited Determination**, the QIO must notify the beneficiary, the beneficiary's physician and the HHA of the QIO's determination as to whether the **termination** by the HHA was a correct decision. The QIO's notification may be by telephone followed by a written notice.

    The QIO's notice of its determination should set forth the rationale for the determination, and the beneficiary's rights to a **Expedited Reconsideration** by the **QIC** of the QIO's determination including information about how to request such **Reconsideration**.

(c)   **Expedited Reconsideration**.

- The beneficiary has the right to **Expedited Reconsideration** by an appropriate **Qualified Independent Contractor** (QIC) of the QIO's Expedited Determination. A beneficiary who wishes to obtain **Expedited Reconsideration** must submit a request in the Reconsideration to the appropriate **QIC**, in writing or by telephone, no later than noon of the calendar day following the receipt of the QIO's notice of termination.

- On the day the **QIC** receives a request for an **Expedited Determination**, it must immediately notify the QIO and the HHA of the request by the beneficiary for an **Expedited Reconsideration**.

- No later than seventy-two (72) hours after receipt of the request for **Expedited Reconsideration**, the **QIC** must notify the QIO, the beneficiary, the beneficiary's physician, and the HHA of its decision. The QIC's initial notification may be done by telephone, followed by written notice (**QIC Notice**). The **QIC Notice** will set forth the rationale for the QIC's decision, and information about the beneficiary's right to further appeal.

VI. WHEN DOES MEDICARE CONSIDER IT IS A SECONDARY PAYER AND ANOTHER PLAN COVERING THE MEDICARE BENEFICIARY IS THE PRIMARY PAYER?

When another health plan covers benefits for a plan participant who is also a Medicare beneficiary entitled to such benefits under Medicare **Part A** and/or **Part B**, Medicare considers that such other plan is the **primary payer** for the benefits and that Medicare is only the **secondary payer** in such cases. Accordingly, should Medicare make payment for the benefits that should have been made by **primary payer**, Medicare may obtain recovery against the **primary payer**. Medicare is empowered to recover payments it incorrectly made if recovery is sought within three (3) years after the rendition of the services covered by the payment. Medicare may make conditional payments under the Medicare **secondary payer** provisions if a **primary plan** such as a group health plan, or a workmen's compensation plan, has not made or cannot reasonably be expected to promptly make payment; any such payment is conditional on reimbursement to Medicare by the **primary plan**. The Federal government may bring an action against any and all entities responsible for payment under a primary plan. When such conditional payment is made, the government may receive double damages under such circumstances.

VII. WHAT IS THE PROGRAM FOR ALL-INCLUSIVE HOME CARE OF THE ELDERLY (PACE)?

This program began as a **Medicare** <u>and</u> **Medicaid** demonstration project initially tested at ten sites and eventually became an <u>option open to all states</u>. PACE targets frail elderly persons living at home who are eligible for nursing home care. The program integrates health and **long-term care** services in an **adult day care** setting and uses a multidisciplinary **case management** team of providers, including physicians, nurses, social workers, nutritionists, occupational and speech therapists, and health and transportation personnel. PACE participants are required to attend an **adult day care** center regularly.

The **Balanced Budget Act** of 1997 established PACE as a state option to furnish comprehensive health care to persons who are enrolled with an organization that has contracted to operate the PACE program, who are eligible for **Medicaid**, and who receive **Medicaid** solely through the PACE program.

Chapter 3

PACE
(continued)

PACE providers may be public or private not-for-profit entities. The salient characteristics of PACE offered as a state option are set forth below.

— Persons eligible for PACE must be fifty-five (55) years of age or older; require nursing facility level of care that would be covered under a state's **Medicaid** program; reside in the service area of the PACE program; and meet such other eligibility conditions as may be imposed under the PACE program agreement. Eligible individuals include both Medicare and Medicaid beneficiaries. Medicare participants not enrolled in the PACE program through Medicaid must pay **premiums** equal to Medicaid capitation. PACE enrollees will be reevaluated annually to determine if they continue to need nursing facility level of care.

— Under a PACE agreement, a provider at a minimum must provide eligible persons all care and services covered under Medicare and Medicaid. The services must be provided without any limitation or condition as to amount, duration and scope and without application of **deductibles**, **co-payments**, **coinsurance** or other cost-sharing that would otherwise apply under Medicare or Medicaid. The services must be provided twenty-four (24) hours per day, every day of the year through a comprehensive multi-disciplinary health and social services delivery system which integrates **acute** and **long-term care** services.

— Primary medical care for a PACE enrollee must be furnished by a **primary care physician** who serves as a gatekeeper for access to treatment by specialists. **CMS** may grant waivers of this requirement. A **primary care physician**, registered nurse, medical director, program director, other health professionals and a governing body to guide the operation must be part of the multi-disciplinary team.

VIII. CAN A PHYSICIAN OPT OUT OF MEDICARE?

Yes.

Physicians and certain other practitioners can opt out of Medicare, and ask their Medicare patients to sign **private contracts** if beneficiaries want to receive these services. The providers who enter into such contracts include doctors of medicine and osteopathy, podiatrists, dentists, optometrists, clinical social workers, clinical psychiatrists, physicians' assistants, nurse practitioners, clinical nurse practitioners, clinical nurse specialists, certified nurses, nurse anesthetists and certified nurse midwives. These private contracts are treated as outside the Medicare system. As such, a physician or practitioner may not receive from Medicare, or from an organization that receives Medicare reimbursement, any payment for any item or services furnished to a patient. In other words, Medicare will not pay nor reimburse, directly or indirectly, for health services under a private contract.

Private contracts are **subject to the requirements which are set forth in Appendix G**.

Chapter 3   Coordination of Medicare and Employer Plans

IX. IS THERE ANY COORDINATION OF COVERAGE BETWEEN MEDICARE AND EMPLOYER PLANS?

Yes.

A. What Is the Coverage Coordination for Employees Age 65 or Older?

Employer group health plans or Medicare group health plans of employers with twenty (20) or more employees, are required to offer to Medicare-eligibles age 65 or over and working spouses who are age 65 or over, the same health insurance benefit under the same conditions offered to younger workers and spouses. In such situations the beneficiary's **spouse** has the option to accept or reject the **employer's health plan**. If an employee accepts the **employer's health plan**, it will be the first payer of an employee's health claims. Medicare will become the **secondary payer**. If the beneficiary rejects the employer health plan, Medicare will remain the primary health insurance payer. If an employee elects Medicare to be the **primary payer**, the employer cannot offer coverage that supplements Medicare.

B. What Is the Coverage Coordination for Retired Medicare-eligible Employees?

Many companies provide health insurance benefits to their Medicare-eligible retirees as part of the company retirement package. **In order to avoid a duplication or overlapping between benefits of a company plan and Medicare, the plans often coordinate the two sets of benefits by provision in the company plan for carve-out coverage, wrap-around coverage, coordination of benefits coverage and exclusion coverage** (see Appendix H).

X. MAY EMPLOYEES, WHEN THEIR EMPLOYMENT IS TERMINATED, HAVE CONTINUING MEDICAL SERVICES UNDER THEIR PREVIOUS EMPLOYER'S MEDICAL INSURANCE PLAN?

Yes.

The **Consolidated Omnibus Budget Reconciliation Act (COBRA) of 1985** requires that the employer continue to provide medical insurance to an employee for a specified time (e.g., eighteen (18) months if the employee's services were terminated) after the employee has left his/her employment. The **COBRA coverage** is for medical insurance that the employer then has in effect, and is at the employee's sole expense.

If a Medicare eligible has **COBRA coverage** when he/she first enrolls in Medicare, the coverage may end. The employer has the option of canceling the coverage if the first enrollment in Medicare is after the date the employee elected the **COBRA coverage**. Alternatively, after the employee attains age 65 or older, and he/she has **COBRA coverage**, the **employer group plan** may require the Medicare eligible to sign up for **Part B**.

XI. WILL MEDICARE HELP PAY FOR OTHER SERVICES INCIDENTAL TO OR SUPPLEMENTAL TO HOME CARE?

Yes. They are services and supplies covered by Medicare Part B.

A. What Are the Covered Outpatient Services?

- Services of physicians (including diagnosis, therapy, consultations and home, office and institutional calls), surgeons, pathologists, radiologists, anesthesiologists and osteopaths, and services of certain non-physician health care practitioners which are incidental to the services of a physician.

    [**Before any surgery,** Medicare recommends an **opinion from a second doctor** to help clarify the patient's decision. Medicare will help pay for both a second and, if necessary, a third opinion, if the first and **second opinions** contradict each other.]

- Physicians' assistants, nurse practitioners, clinical nurse specialists, certified nurse midwives, clinical psychologists, clinical social workers, physical therapists and occupational therapists.

- Services by **chiropractors** with respect to treatment of **subluxation** (i.e., partial dislocation) of the spine by means of manual manipulation. (Medicare will not pay for any other diagnostic or therapeutic services by chiropractors, excluding **x-rays**).

- Fees of **podiatrists**, including the treatment of plantar warts, but not for routine foot care.

- The cost of **diagnosis and treatment of eye and ear ailments**, including treatment of aphasia.

- **Plastic surgery for repair of an accidental injury**, an impaired limb or a malformed part of the body.

- **Radiological or pathological services** furnished by a physician to a hospital in-patient.

Chapter 3

Part B Outpatient Services (continued)

- The cost of **blood-clotting factors** and supplies necessary for the self-administration of the clotting factors, for **hemophiliac patients**.

- **Immunosuppressive drugs** used in the first three (3) years after transplantation, plus an extension of up to eight (8) additional months.

- **Outpatient physical and occupational therapy and speech-language pathology services.** (See Appendix A)

- **Outpatient hospital services.** (See Appendix B)

- **Outpatient mental health services** furnished by hospital outpatient units and qualified community health services. (See Appendix C)

- **Radiation therapy** with **x-ray**, radium or radioactive isotopes.

- **Surgical dressings, splints, casts and other devices for reduction of fractures and dislocations.**

- **Rental or purchase of durable medical equipment**, such as **iron lungs, oxygen tents, hospital beds** and **wheelchairs** for use in the patient's home; **prosthetic devices**, such as artificial heart valves or synthetic arteries, designed to replace part or all of an internal organ (but not **false teeth, hearing aids** or **eyeglasses**); **braces, artificial** limbs, **artificial** eyes. (See Appendix D)

- **Ambulance service to and from the hospital, nursing home and the patient's home** if the patient's condition does not permit the use of other methods of transportation. (See Appendix E)

- **Certain costs relating to diabetes:** The cost of **training services** (including the skills of self-administrative **injection drugs**) **in an ambulatory setting for diabetes outpatient self-management**, if recommended by a physician; a blood glucose lancet monitor and, every three (3) months, one hundred (100) lancets plus one-hundred (100) test strips. [See medical nutrition therapy under "kidneys" below.]

- **The following costs relative to kidneys:**

    - Kidney **dialysis equipment** and necessary supplies.

    - The cost of care for kidney donors including all reasonable preparatory, operation and post-operation recovery expenses associated with the donation, without regard to the usual Medicare **deductibles**, **coinsurance** and **premium** payment.

    - The costs of all supplies and equipment, including portable equipment, necessary to perform **home dialysis**.

    - The costs of **monitoring** the patient's home adaptation; visits by qualified provider or facility personnel **in accordance with the plan prepared and periodically reviewed by a professional team;** installation and maintenance of **dialysis** equipment and testing; and treatment of the water.

    - The costs of **medical nutrition therapy** services for individuals who have **diabetes** or kidney disease unless on **dialysis**) with a physician's referral. These services are covered for three (3) years after a **kidney transplant**.

- **Transplants.** **Heart transplants** when performed in specialized facilities by trained personnel, and **liver and lung transplants**.

- The cost of a **flu shot** each fall, and one **pneumonia** shot per lifetime. Neither the $135 annual (2008) **deductible** nor the twenty (20) percent **coinsurance** applies to the pneumonia shot.

- The cost of **hepatitis B vaccine** for high and intermediate-risk individuals when it is administered in a hospital or renal **dialysis** facility.

- Screening **tests, as a preventative of disease.** (See Appendix F)

- The cost of an **injectable drug approved for the treatment of a bone fracture related to post-menopausal osteoporosis** under the following conditions: the patient's attending physician certifies the patient is unable to learn the skills needed to self-administer, or is physically or mentally incapable of self-administering the drug; and the patient meets the requirements for Medicare coverage of **home health services**.

- One pair of **eyeglasses** following **cataract surgery**.

- The cost of **bone mass measurements** for women over age 65 who are at high risk for **osteoporosis**, and for beneficiaries with vertebral abnormalities and certain bone defects.

- **Intravenous immune gobulin** for treatment of primary immune deficiency diseases when medically necessary.

- **Diagnostic x-ray tests, diagnostic laboratory tests, and other** diagnostic **tests** are covered by **Medicare Part B** and are not subject to the payment of any **deductible** or **coinsurance**. The tests must be ordered by the physician who is treating the beneficiary. The tests may be provided by an independent laboratory which must accept assignment for the test.

- **Psychiatric care.** Medicare helps pay for services received for non-hospital treatment of **mental illness**. This includes services from doctors, comprehensive outpatient rehabilitation facilities, physician assistants, psychologists and clinical social workers. Services for non-hospital treatment of a mental illness are subject to a special payment rule: Once the annual **deductible** is met, **Medicare Part B** pays only fifty (50) percent of approved charges for these services, not the eighty (80) percent customary for other services. Partial

Chapter 3

Part B Outpatient Services
(continued)

hospitalization services for treatment of **mental illness** are not subject to this special payment rule.

- **Emergency hospital care.** Federal law requires hospitals that participate in Medicare and have an emergency room to examine all persons seeking care in the emergency room to determine whether they have an emergency medical condition. If staff personnel determine that an emergency condition exists, they must provide stabilizing treatment that is requisite medical treatment so that when the person is transferred from the hospital, no deterioration of the person's condition is likely to result.

B. **For Which Outpatient Services Will Medicare Part B Not Pay?**

1. **Exclusions.**

    1.1 **General**. The two largest Medicare **exclusions** that may affect most people are **prescription drug coverage** (except as mentioned above), and **long-term care** (**especially custodial care**, in a nursing home or at home). Since most **long-term care** needs are **custodial**, Medicare therefore does not cover most **long-term care**.

    1.2 **Express Exclusions**. Medicare expressly excludes coverage of many services:

    — **full-time nursing care;**

    — **routine foot care, or orthopedic shoes;**

    — **meals** delivered to the home;

    — **cosmetic surgery;**

    — **homemaker chores** (e.g., general housekeeping, meal preparation, shopping) unrelated to patient care;

    — **custodial care;**

    — services that would not be covered as **in-patient hospital services;**

    — **routine physical examinations**, and tests directly related to such examinations (except some **Pap smears**, **mammograms**, and **prostate cancer** and other specified screenings);

— eye **(optometrists)** or ear examinations to prescribe or fit **eyeglasses** or **hearing aids**;

— **immunizations**, except **flu** vaccinations, **pneumococcal pneumonia** and **hepatitis B vaccinations**, or immunizations required because of any injury or immediate risk of infection;

— **acupuncture**;

— most **chiropractic** services;

— **dental care**;

— **private room**, TV and radio;

— **private nurses**;

— **services payable by workers compensation, auto insurance, employer health plan or other governmental programs**; and

— **services provided outside the United States.**

1.3 **Reasonable and Necessary Requirement Exclusion.** Medicare excludes any services that are not "**reasonable and necessary**" for the diagnosis or treatment of illness or injury, or to improve the functioning of a malformed body organ. There are no judicial decisions interpreting this term. However, the legislative history and Medicare manuals recognize that **reasonable and necessary** care needs to be practical and individualized. CMS in turn has established many policies applying the general exclusion provision, frequently referred to as the "**medical necessity**" **exclusion**. Further, Medicare coverage decisions relating to this exclusion frequently are made on a case-by-case basis by Medicare carriers and intermediaries and by providers of health services.

Chapter 3   Part B Outpatient Services (continued)

C. **Are There Cost-sharing Expenses, Deductibles, Premiums, Coinsurance for Part B Services?**

Yes. They are set forth below.

1. **Annual Part B Deductible.**

This **deductible** of $135 (2008) must be paid by Medicare-eligibles enrolled in **Part B**.

2. **Part B Coinsurance (Co-Payments).**

Generally, equal to twenty (20) percent of Medicare's **Maximum Approved Charges** for Medicare-covered services, (including **durable medical equipment**) must be paid by Medicare-eligibles (a different percentage applies to certain services as set forth in Chapter 3 section XI.A) and in certain of the appendices to Chapter 3).

Note: The deductibles, coinsurance and co-payments represent so-called "gaps" in Medicare coverage. To fill these gaps (i.e., the difference between the amount paid by Medicare and the Medicare-approved charges), Medicare-eligibles may obtain private **Medigap** insurance policies to protect against these areas in which the Medicare program is deficient in coverage.

3. **Premiums.**

Individuals age 65 or older, who are entitled to **Social Security** retirement or **Railroad Retirement** benefits generally are entitled to **Part A** benefits without payment of premiums. (Persons not entitled to **Part A** benefits may be able to purchase them.)

The monthly premium required to be paid by beneficiaries enrolled in **Part B** is $96.40 in 2008, with a **surcharge** for higher-income beneficiaries. <u>The premiums are set forth in the table below</u>:

Chapter 3   **Part B Outpatient Services**
                                                                                                        (continued)

Yearly Income		Monthly Premium (2008)
Individual Tax Return	Joint Tax Return	
$82,000 or below	$164,000 or below	$ 96.40
$82,001 - $102,000	$164,001 - $204,000	$122.20
$102,001 - $153,000	$204,001 - $306,000	$160.90
$153,001 - $205,000	$306,001 - $410,000	$199.70
Above $205,000	Above $410,000	$238.40

    D.   **What Is the Billing and Payment Process for Part B Services and Supplies?**

        1.   **Billing.**

A claim (**bill**) for payment may be submitted to the carrier by physicians, practitioners, medical suppliers either on their own behalf for payment to them, or on behalf of the beneficiary for payment to him/her, depending upon whether the provider has entered into a Participation Agreement with Medicare to accept **Assignment** by the beneficiary or not. A provider who agrees to accept assignment is known as a **participating provider**.

        (a)   **Where provider has accepted assignment.** The beneficiary, by signing an assignment statement, will assign to a provider his/her right to payment for services rendered and supplies provided, and authorize payment by Medicare to the provider. Medicare will pay eighty (80) percent of the **Medicare-approved (allowed) charges** to the provider. <u>By accepting **assignment**, the provider agrees to accept the amount approved by Medicare as the full charge for the services and items rendered and supplied</u>.

        (b)   **Where provider has not accepted assignment (Assignment of Services).** Although payment is made to the beneficiary, the provider is responsible for handling, on the beneficiary's behalf, the paper work of claims to Medicare for payment. The provider will bill and seek payment from the beneficiary on the basis of an itemized bill. This method of billing is known as **Balance Billing**. <u>Payment will be made by Medicare to the beneficiary for eighty (80) percent of the **Medicare-approved charge**. The beneficiary is responsible for paying the bill which amount may not legally exceeds one-hundred fifteen (115) percent of the Medicare-approved Charge.</u> This **approved charge** is known as the **limiting charge** or **actual charge**. Several states by statute have prohibited (or limited) **balance billing**, and thus in effect have mandated **assignment**.

2. **Payment of Bills.**

(a) In the case of services rendered under Part B <u>by an institutional provider</u> (e.g., home health agencies), **payments are made by Medicare directly to the provider. The provider in turn may then charge the beneficiary for applicable deductibles and coinsurance payments**.

(b) In the case of services rendered under Part B <u>by physicians, practitioners, durable equipment suppliers</u>, **payment may be made by Medicare to the physician or other providers only if the right to payment is assigned to them by the beneficiary and if they agree to be paid according to the rules of Assignment (as set forth in section D.1(a) above).**

E. Are There Special Rates for the Payment of Part B Services and Supplies to Low-income Beneficiaries?

Yes. **Medicaid** will pay for certain Medicare benefits (**deductibles, co-payments, coinsurance**, and/or **premiums**) for **low-income Medicare beneficiaries**, as set forth below:

1. **Qualified Medicare Beneficiary (QMB).**

Chapter 3

Part B Outpatient Services
(continued)

Federal law requires state **Medicaid** programs to **buy-in** Medicare coverage for certain low-income Medicare beneficiaries. The buy-in consists of <u>payment of deductibles and coinsurance</u> costs under Medicare **Part A** and **Part B**, payment of premiums under **Part B**, and payment of premiums under **Part A** for those not entitled to **Part A** by virtue of receiving Social Security benefits. These beneficiaries are known as **Qualified Medicare Beneficiaries** (QMB).

QMBs must:

— meet federally prescribed income and resource standards. Individuals must have incomes below one-hundred (100) percent of the **Federal poverty level**, and their non-exempt resources cannot exceed twice the **Supplemental Security Income** (SSI) resource standard ($4,000 for an individual and $6,000 for a family of two). The poverty level in 2008 is $10,400 for an individual and $14,000 for a couple.

— be entitled to Part A hospitalization. If they otherwise would be eligible for **QMB** benefits but are not automatically eligible for Medicare **Part A**, the state must pay their **Part A premiums** to make them eligible for **Part A**.

[A subset of **QMBs** is known as **Dual Eligibles**. They are individuals whose income is <u>below one-hundred (100) percent of</u> the **Federal poverty level** and who have low assets and are eligible for full coverage under both Medicare and **Medicaid**. They are exempt from mandatory enrollment in **Medicaid managed care**. The state Medicaid program pays the Medicare Part B **premiums** for **dual eligibles** and should also pay Medicare **Part A premiums** for those not entitled to **Part A** by virtue of receiving **Social Security** retirement benefits. All **dual eligibles** are QMBs. They are entitled to the full spectrum of both **Medicaid** and Medicare benefits.]

2. **Specified Low-income Medicare Beneficiary (SLMB).**

Chapter 3   **Part B Outpatient Services**
                                            (continued)

An individual entitled to Medicare **Part A** benefits, whose income is <u>between one-hundred (100) percent and one-hundred twenty (120) percent</u> of **Federal poverty** guidelines and whose **non-exempt resources** are $4,000 or less ($6,000 in the case of a couple), is eligible to have **Medicaid** pay his/her Medicare **Part B** <u>premium</u>. This individual is referred to as a SLMB. As with the QMB program, the **SLMB** program is managed by the state agency that provides medical assistance under **Medicaid**.

3. **Low-income Qualifying Individual (QI-1).**

   An individual is selected by the state as a qualifying individual (QI-1). A QI-1 is an individual who meets the QMB criteria, except that his/her income level is <u>at least one-hundred twenty (120) percent but less than one-hundred thirty-five (135) percent</u> of the **Federal poverty level** for a family of the size involved and his/her **non-exempt resources** are $4,000 or less ($6,000 in the case of a couple). There is no resource limit in New York State and some other states for this program. The state is required to pay the full amount of the Medicare **Part B premiums** of such a qualifying individual (but only for premiums payable during a statutorily prescribed period). However, the individual cannot be otherwise eligible for medical assistance under the state-approved plan.

4. **Qualified Disabled and Working Individual (QDWI).**

   State **Medicaid** programs must pay Medicare **Part A premiums** for individuals whose income is <u>below two-hundred (200) percent</u> of the **Federal poverty level;** who are entitled to Medicare on the basis of **disability**; who are in a trial work period and are entitled to continue Medicare coverage while they are in that work period; whose resources do not exceed twice SSI resource levels ($4,000 for individuals, and $6,000 in the case of couples); and who are not otherwise eligible for **Medicaid**. They are not entitled to other Medicaid services.

Long-term Care at Home Consumer Guide

APPENDIX A

OUTPATIENT SKILLED THERAPY

Generally Medicare will pay for **outpatient physical and occupational therapy**, including **speech-language pathology** services, received as part of a patient's treatment in a doctor's office or as an outpatient of a participating hospital, **skilled nursing facility**, or through a **home health agency**, approved clinic, rehabilitative agency or public health agency. The services must be furnished under a plan established by a physician or therapist, and the conditions set forth in sections I – IV below must be satisfied. Further, payment for the services must be made as specified in sections V and VI below.

I. HOMEBOUND NOT A REQUIREMENT

Skilled therapy services may be furnished to a Medicare beneficiary, whether or not **homebound**, on an outpatient basis by a participating hospital, **skilled nursing facility**, clinic, rehabilitation center, **comprehensive outpatient rehabilitation facility**, public health agency, or also, if the beneficiary is **homebound**, by a **home health agency**. The provided services are covered as one of the medical and other health services, under Medicare **Part B**.

Instead of obtaining skilled therapy services from a participating Medicare facility, patients can receive services directly from private practicing, Medicare-approved therapists performing such services **in their office or in the patient's home, if such treatment is prescribed by a doctor**.

II. REASONABLE AND NECESSARY REQUIREMENT

The therapy services, to be covered by Medicare, must be **reasonable and necessary**. To be considered such, the service must be a specific, safe and effective treatment for the beneficiary's condition. The required service(s) must be sufficiently complex or the condition of the beneficiary such that the services can be performed only by a qualified therapist. There also must be an expectation that the beneficiary's condition will improve materially in a reasonably predictable period of time or that such services are necessary to establish a safe maintenance program. The services must relate directly and specifically to a treatment regimen established by a physician, after any needed consultation with the qualified therapist, and designed to treat the beneficiary's illness or injury. The **therapy services** cannot merely relate to activities for the general physical welfare of the beneficiary.

III. PHYSICIAN'S CARE PLAN AND CERTIFICATION

In addition to being **reasonable and necessary**, outpatient therapy services must meet the following conditions:

— The outpatient must be under the care of a physician.

— Services must be furnished and related directly to and specifically under a written **plan of care** established by a physician or the therapist who will provide the **therapy services**. The plan must be established before the treatment is begun and reviewed by the attending physician in consultation with the therapist at least every thirty (30) days.

— The physician must certify at intervals of at least every thirty (30) days that a continuing need exists for such services and should estimate how long the services will be needed.

— Recertification should be obtained at the time the plan of treatment is reviewed.

IV. APPLICABLE STANDARDS

Medicare will not make payment for **outpatient occupational therapy** services or **outpatient physical therapy**, furnished as an incident to a physician's professional services that do not meet the standards applicable to a therapist furnishing such services in a clinic, rehabilitation agency or public health agency.

V. AMOUNT OF PAYMENT BY PATIENT

The provider of **therapy services**, other than a hospital outpatient department, may charge the patient any part of the Medicare **Part B** $135 (2008) annual **deductible** not met, and the twenty (20) percent **co-payment** of the **Medicare-approved charge**. However, if an individual receives outpatient services at a hospital outpatient department, as opposed to the other settings, his/her **co-payment** is twenty (20) percent of the hospital bill – a much higher amount than the standard **co-payment** of twenty (20) percent of the Medicare-approved charge. However, this disparity gradually will diminish so that the twenty (20) percent **co-payment** of the hospital bill gradually will equal the standard **co-payment**.

Chapter 3   **Appendix A Outpatient Skilled Therapy (continued)**

VI. FINANCIAL LIMITATIONS (CAP)

Until December 31, 2001, payments by Medicare to beneficiaries for **outpatient physical therapy services**, which includes **speech-language pathology**, were not subject to any **charge limit**. Beginning in 2002, an annual limit of $1,500 was applied to all outpatient **physical therapy services**, including **speech language pathology**, excepting services in a hospital outpatient department (which has no cap). A separate $1500 limitation applied to **occupational therapy**. Thereafter these limitations were suspended for the period between December 8, 2003 and December 31, 2005; the suspension ended on December 31, 2005. **Financial limitations on outpatient therapy services resumed on those services effective January 1, 2006. The annual limit on the allowed amount for outpatient physical therapy and speech pathology combined is $1,810 (2008); the limit for occupational therapy is $1,810 (2008). The limits apply to outpatient Part B therapy services from all settings except outpatient hospital services and hospital emergency rooms.**

VII. TYPES OF THERAPISTS

The types of therapists are set forth below:

— **Physical Therapist**. A physical therapist has a bachelor degree and also some postgraduate training. **Physical therapy** is frequently needed by a patient who has lost some use of his or her limbs or muscles because of an illness or accident.

After reviewing the physician's medical diagnosis and treatment plan, a **physical therapist** may visit the patient at home, as required under a **plan of care**. The therapist generally prepares a treatment schedule and visits the patient on a routine basis until determining, after consultation with the physician that therapy is no longer necessary or advisable.

— **Speech-language Pathologist**. A **speech-language pathologist** has a graduate degree and is certified by the American Speech Language Hearing Association. A **speech-language pathologist** can assess the patient's problem, design a treatment program, and provide therapy to help the patient regain or maintain speech or language skills.

— **Occupational Therapist**. An **occupational therapist** has either a bachelor's or master's degree with special training in **occupational therapy**. Such a therapist may be needed by a patient who has suffered an illness or injury which has affected daily activities,

Chapter 3 — Appendix A Outpatient Skilled Therapy (continued)

movement or perceptual abilities. The **occupational therapist** evaluates the patient's ability to **dress**, wash, walk or perform other routine functions and, when necessary, provides devices which add to the patient's comfort. Examples include using larger buttons on clothes to facilitate **dressing**; adding a board to the arm of **wheelchair** to help support a patient's paralyzed arm; and providing a leg or ankle splint to aid in walking.

APPENDIX B

OUTPATIENT DEPARTMENT HOSPITAL SERVICES

Medicare **Part B** helps pay for the following **outpatient department hospital services**:

- **Blood transfusions** furnished to a person as an outpatient;
- **Drugs** and **biologicals** that cannot be self-administered;
- **Laboratory tests** billed by the hospital;
- **Mental health care** if a physician certifies that in-patient treatment would be required without it;
- Medical supplies such as **splints** and **casts**;
- Services in an **emergency room** or outpatient clinic, including same day surgery; and
- **X-rays** and other **radiology services** billed by a hospital

If an individual receives **outpatient department (OPD) services** at a hospital, other than for **mental health**, he/she is responsible for paying twenty (20) percent of whatever the hospital charges not to exceed the standard Medicare hospital in-patient **deductible** – not merely the customary and lesser twenty (20) percent of the **Medicare-approved amount** for **Part B** services rendered in other settings. According to **CMS** rules issued as a result of the **Balanced Budget Act of 1997**, this disparity in the amount of **coinsurance** for OPD services is scheduled to diminish gradually and become the same as the standard **co-payment**. Under these rules, the **co-payment** for **hospital OPD services** is subject to a cap equal to the hospital in-patient **deductible** ($1,024 in 2008).

If an individual receives **outpatient mental health services**, his/her **coinsurance** share is fifty (50) percent of the **Medicare-approved amount**.

APPENDIX C

MENTAL HEALTH SERVICES FURNISHED BY HOSPITAL OUTPATIENT UNITS AND QUALIFIED COMMUNITY MENTAL HEALTH CENTERS

Under certain conditions, Medicare **Part B** helps to pay for partial hospitalization for **mental health services** furnished by a hospital outpatient unit and by qualified **community mental health centers**. Partial hospitalization means an ambulatory program of active care that lasts less than twenty-four (24) hours a day. In addition, Medicare helps to pay for services received for non-hospital treatment of **mental illness**. This includes services from doctors, **comprehensive outpatient rehabilitation facilities**, physician assistants, psychologists and clinical social workers. Services for non-hospital treatment of **mental illness** are subject to a special payment rule. Once the **annual deductible** is met, Medicare Part B pays only fifty (50) percent of approved charges for these services, not the customary eighty (80) percent for other services. Partial hospitalization services for treatment of **mental illness** are not subject to this special payment rule.

APPENDIX D

DURABLE MEDICAL EQUIPMENT

Durable medical equipment (DME) is furnished to a beneficiary for use in the patient's home and is covered under **Part B**, whether furnished on a rental basis or purchased.

I. DEFINITION OF DURABLE MEDICAL EQUIPMENT

DME is equipment that: (1) can withstand repeated use, (2) is primarily and customarily used to serve a medical purpose, (3) generally is not useful to a person in the absence of illness or injury and (4) is appropriate to use in the home.

A. Durability. An item is considered durable if it can withstand repeated use (i.e., the type of equipment that normally could be rented). Medical supplies with expendable nature such as the catheters and bandages are not considered to be durable equipment. Other items, though they may be durable in nature, may fall into other Medicare coverage categories such as braces, prosthetic devices, or artificial arms, legs and eyes.

B. Medical Equipment. An item is considered medical equipment if it is primarily and customarily used for medical purposes and is not generally useful in the absence of illness or injury (e.g., hospital beds, wheelchairs, hemodialysis equipment, iron lung respirators, intermittent positive fresh breathing machines, medical regulators, oxygen tents, crutches, canes, trapeze bars, walkers, inhalators, nebulizers, commodes, suction machines, and traction equipment). Seat-lift chairs are covered only for the seat-lift mechanism, not for the chair itself. The following items are excluded from coverage as DME when furnished by a home health agency: (1) intraocular lenses and (2) medical supplies (including canisters, catheter supplies, ostomy bags and supplies related to ostomy care).

<u>Note:</u> Conditions of coverage are contained in the *Medicare Issuers Manual*. Certain items such as bathroom grab bars are not DME.

II. REQUIREMENTS FOR COVERAGE

A. Use in Patient's Home. An item of DME must be used in the patient's home in order to be covered for purposes of rental or purchase of DME.

A patient's home may be: patient's own dwelling and apartment, a relative's home, a home for the aged or some other type of institution. Neither a hospital nor a skilled nursing facility may be considered a patient's home.

B. Necessary and Reasonable. Coverage is subject to the requirement that the equipment be reasonable and necessary for treating illness or injury or improving the functioning of a body member.

C. Prescription. Medicare requires a physician's prescription for DME, prosthetics or products and other supplies.

D. Certificate of Medical Necessity (CMN). For DME items or services billed to Medicare, the **supplier** must receive a signed Certificate of Medical Necessity from the treating physician. The CMN can serve as the physician's order if the narrative description is sufficiently detailed.

III. REPAIRS, MAINTENANCE, REPLACEMENT AND DELIVERY.

Medicare may pay for the repair, maintenance, and replacement of medically required DME that the beneficiary owns or is purchasing, including the equipment which has been in use before the user enrolled in Medicare **Part B**.

A. Repairs. Repairs to equipment that beneficiary is purchasing or already owns are covered when necessary to make the equipment serviceable. The expense of repairs may not exceed the estimated expense of purchasing or renting another item of equipment.

B. Maintenance. Medicare pays for maintenance and servicing of DME in the following categories: inexpensive or frequently purchased items, customized items, other **prosthetic** and **orthotic devices**, and capped rental items. Maintenance and service of items, which frequently require substantial servicing for **oxygen equipment,** are not reimbursed. Routine periodic servicing such as testing, cleaning, regulating and checking of the beneficiary's equipment is not covered.

C. Replacement. Replacement is covered in the case of loss, irreparable damage, or when required, should there be a change in the person's condition.

D. Delivery. Delivery and service charges are covered.

Chapter 3   **Appendix D Durable Medical Equipment**
(continued)

IV. SUPPLIES AND ACCESSORIES

Reimbursement may be made for supplies, for example, **oxygen** necessary for the effective use of **DME**. Such supplies include those **drug** and **biologicals** that must be put directly into the equipment in order for the achieved therapeutic benefit of the **DME** or to insure the proper functioning of the equipment.

V. OXYGEN SERVICES IN THE HOME

Oxygen and oxygen equipment provided in the home are covered by Medicare. Initial claims for **oxygen services** must include a completed **certificate of medical necessity** to establish where the coverage criteria are met and to insure the **oxygen services** are provided consistent with the prescription order or other medical documentation.

VI. PURCHASE OPTION FOR CAPPED RENTAL ITEMS

In the category of capped rental items (i.e., the rental may not exceed the monthly fee schedule amounts prescribed by Medicare), Medicare must offer a Medicare beneficiary an option to purchase these items. Beneficiaries have one month from the date the supplier makes the offer to accept the purchase option. For **power-driven wheelchairs** the supplier must also make permissible a purchase option to beneficiaries at the time the equipment is initially furnished.

VII. PROSTHETIC DEVICES (OTHER THAN DENTAL)

Prosthetic devices (other than dental) that replace all or part of an internal body organ or replace all or part of the function of a permanently inoperative or malfunctioning internal body organ are covered by Medicare when furnished incident to a physician's services or on a physician's order.

    A. Examples of Prosthetic Devices. Artificial limbs, parenteral and enteral nutrition, cardiac **pacemakers**, prosthetic lenses, breast prostheses (including a surgical brassiere) for post-mastectomy patients, maxillo-facial devices and devices that replace all or part of the ear or nose. Chucks, diapers, rubber sheets, etc. are supplies that are not covered. **Colostomy** (and other **ostomy**) bags and other items supplied directly for **ostomy care** are covered as **prosthetic devices**.

    B. Prosthetic Lenses. The term "internal body organ" includes the lens of an **eye**. **Prostheses** replacing the lens of an eye include post-surgical lenses customarily used during convalescence from eye surgery in which the lens of the eye was removed. In addition, permanent lenses also are covered when required by the individual lacking the organic lens of the eye because of surgical removal or congenital absence.

C. Dentures. Dentures are excluded from coverage. However, when a denture or a portion of the denture is an integral part (built-in) of a covered prosthesis (e.g., an obturator to fill an opening in the palate), it is covered as part of that prosthetic.

D. Supplies, Repairs, Adjustments, and Replacements. Medicare covers supplies that are necessary for the effective use of a **prosthetic device** (e.g., the batteries needed to operate an artificial larynx). Adjustment of prosthetic devices required by wear or by a change in the patient's condition is covered when ordered by a physician. Replacement of conventional **eyeglasses** or contact lenses is not covered.

Necessary supplies, adjustments, repairs, and replacements are covered even when the device had been in use before the user enrolled in **Part B** of the program, so long as the device continues to be medically required.

APPENDIX E

AMBULANCE TRANSPORTATION

Transportation by ambulance of a Medicare beneficiary who is receiving Part A benefits while a patient at a hospital, **critical access hospital (CAH)** or **skilled nursing facility (SNF)** is covered by **Part A**.

Medicare **Part B** helps pay for medically necessary **ambulance transportation** of a beneficiary who is not a patient of a hospital, CAH or **SNF** but only if the **ambulance**, equipment and personnel meet Medicare requirements, including origin and destination requirements described below, and if transportation in any other vehicle would endanger a patient's health. **Ambulance** use from one's home to a doctor's office is not covered.

For ambulance transportation to be covered by **Part B**, there must be a medical necessity for such transportation, and other requirements need be met also. The medical necessity requirement is met when a beneficiary is unable to get up from bed without assistance, ambulate or sit in a chair or **wheelchair** and when another means of transportation would be contra-indicated. A physician's certificate of medical necessity is required unless the beneficiary resides at home or is a patient of a facility and not under the direct care of a physician.

If the criteria for coverage are met, ambulance service is covered from any point of origin to the nearest hospital, CAH or SNF capable of furnishing the required level and type of care; from a hospital, CAH or SNF to the beneficiary's home; or from a SNF to the nearest supplier of medically necessary services not available at the SNF where the beneficiary resides.

Transportation from the home of a beneficiary receiving renal **dialysis** for treatment of **end-stage renal disease** to the nearest facility providing renal **dialysis** is covered under **Part B**.

APPENDIX F

PREVENTIVE DISEASE MANAGEMENT SERVICES

I. ANNUAL PROSTATE CANCER SCREENING TESTS

Annual prostate cancer screening tests for men age 50 or over, including **digital rectal exam** and **prostate-specific antigen (PSA) blood tests**. Neither the **Part B** $135 (2008) **annual deductible** nor the twenty (20) percent **coinsurance** applies to the **PSA** test, but they do apply to the **digital rectal exam**.

II. SCREENING PAP SMEARS, SCREENING PELVIC EXAM

Screening pap smears for early detection of cervical cancer, under normal circumstances, are covered every two (2) years. The coverage is authorized on a yearly basis for women at high risk of developing cervical or vaginal cancer and for women of child bearing age who have had a negative test in the three (3) preceding years. The **Part B annual deductible** is waived for screening **pap smears** and **pelvic exams**, but the twenty (20) percent **coinsurance** must be paid by the beneficiary.

III. SCREENING MAMMOGRAPHY

Screening mammography is defined as a radiological procedure provided to a woman for the early detection of breast cancer, including a physician's interpretation of the results of the procedure. For women age 40 and over, screening under normal circumstances is covered every twelve (12) months. For women age 30-39, Medicare will help pay for one baseline mammogram. The **Part B annual deductible** is waived, but not the twenty (20) percent **coinsurance** amount.

IV. CARDIOVASCULAR SCREENING BLOOD TESTS

Cardiovascular screening blood tests are available every five (5) years to patients at risk. For these services beneficiaries do not have to meet a **deductible** or co-pay. At-risk individuals eligible for screening include those with hypertension, dislipidemia, obesity or a family history of **diabetes**. This benefit provides blood tests for the early detection of cardiovascular disease or elevated risk of cardiovascular disease by testing total cholesterol levels, high-density lipoprotein, and triglycerides levels. There is no coinsurance or **Part B deductible** requirement for these **lab tests**. For all other tests, the beneficiary must pay twenty

(20) percent of the **Medicare-approved amounts**, after the **Part B deductible is met**.

V. DIABETES SCREENINGS

Diabetes screenings are covered for certain beneficiaries who are considered at high risk for developing the disease. The screenings include a fasting plasma glucose test. Patients who meet the at-risk criteria can be screened up to twice each year and are not be required to meet a **deductible** or co-pay for the tests. There is no coinsurance or Part B deductible for diabetes screening tests. For all other tests and services, a beneficiary must pay twenty (20) percent of the **Medicare-approved amount** after the yearly **Part B deductible**.

VI. COLORECTAL CANCER SCREENING TESTS: FECAL-OCCULT BLOOD TEST, FLEXIBLE SIGMOIDOSCOPY AND COLONOSCOPY.

Medicare covers the following screenings for colorectal cancer:

- **Fecal-occult blood test,** once every twelve (12) months if age 50 or older, at no cost (i.e., no co-pay nor deductible requirement);

- **Flexible sigmoidoscopy** (FSO), once every four-eight (48) months if age 50 or over, or for those not at high risk, one-hundred twenty (120) months after a previous screening colonoscopy;

- **Colonoscopy** (CO) once every one-hundred twenty (120) months (if at high risk, every twenty-four (24) months), or every forty-eight (48) months after a FSO examination. There is no minimum age.

For FSO and CO examinations, a beneficiary must pay twenty (20) percent of the **Medicare-approved amount**, and, in the case of FSO only, not CO, the yearly Part B deductible. If the test is done in a hospital outpatient department, a beneficiary must pay twenty (20) percent of the **Medicare-approved amount** after meeting the yearly Part B deductible.

VII. GLAUCOMA SCREENING

Glaucoma screening is covered once every twelve (12) months for people who are at high risk for glaucoma, including people with diabetes, a family history of glaucoma, or African Americans age fifty (50) or older. The beneficiary must pay twenty (20) percent of the **Medicare-approved amount** after the yearly **Part B deductible**.

VIII. ULTRASOUND SCREENING FOR ABDOMINAL AORTA ANEURISM

Screening for **abdominal aortic aneurisms**, as of January 1, 2007, is covered for Medicare beneficiaries: (i) who receive a referral for an **ultrasound screening** as a result of an initial **Preventive Physical Examination**, (ii) who have not been previously furnished such an ultrasound screening, <u>and</u> (iii) who either have a family history of abdominal aortic aneurisms or manifest risk factors included in a beneficiary category recommended for screening by the United States Preventive Services Task Force. There is no required **Part B deductible**.

IX. PREVENTIVE PHYSICALS

Within six (6) months of first becoming eligible for Medicare, beneficiaries are eligible for, among other things, a "**Welcome to Medicare Physical**," consisting of a comprehensive exam (not including **lab tests**). The initial **preventive physical** also includes education, **counseling**, and referrals to other preventive services. The beneficiary must pay twenty (20) percent of the **Medicare-approved amount** after the yearly Part B deductible is met.

<u>NOTE</u>

(i) Many vascular specialists say two **diagnostic tests** – **carotid ultrasound** and the **ankle-brachial test** – can provide a clear window into artery disease that can lead to strokes, heart attacks and related lethal events. Despite being two decades old, the **carotid ultrasound and ankle-brachial tests** often are overlooked exams. Many general practitioners have not yet embraced the tests, in large part because Medicare and insurers do not pay for them as screening tools. However, if a doctor writes a referral for one based on the patient's risk-factor profile, the cost of the screening if done at a hospital vascular laboratory, usually may be reimbursed by Medicare Part B.

(ii) The **Centers for Medicare & Medicaid Services (CMS)** has expanded Medicare coverage of **positron emission tomography** (PET scan), when used to confirm an **Alzheimer's disease** diagnosis, to include some Medicare beneficiaries with suspected **Alzheimer's disease** and to include other beneficiaries at risk for **Alzheimer's disease** who are enrolled in a large and easily accessible clinical trial. Medicare beneficiaries who meet specific criteria may participate in the clinical trial and receive a PET scan.

APPENDIX G

PRIVATE CONTRACTS

When a physician or other health care provider opts out of Medicare, the beneficiary and the physician/heath care provider may enter into a private contract for medical services (see Chapter 3, section VIII).

I. BENEFICIARY PROTECTIONS

A private contract:

- must be written and signed by the beneficiary before any item or service is provided pursuant to the contract.

- may not be entered into at a time when a beneficiary is facing an emergency or urgent health care situation.

- must fully indicate that a beneficiary, by signing the contract: (i) agrees not to submit a claim to Medicare for services even if they were otherwise covered under Medicare; (ii) agrees to be responsible whether through insurance or otherwise for payment of such items of services and understands that no Medicare reimbursement will be provided; and (iii) acknowledges that: no Medicare **limiting charges** apply (i.e., no limit to **balance billing**); **Medigap** plans do not, and other supplemental insurance plans may not elect not to, make payment for items of services rendered; the Medicare beneficiary has the right to have such items or services provided by other physicians or practitioners for whom Medicare payment will be made.

- must indicate whether the physician or practitioner is excluded from Medicare participation.

II. NO LIMITING CHARGES

Medicare **limiting charges (charge limits)** do not apply to **private contracts**. In other words, there are no **balance billing** restrictions.

III. PHYSICIAN'S OR PRACTITIONER'S REQUIRED AFFIDAVIT

At the time services are provided under a **private contract**, the physician or practitioner must have a signed affidavit in effect. It must state that the physician or practitioner will not submit any Medicare claim for any item or service provided to any Medicare beneficiary, and will not receive any reimbursement for any such item of service, for a two- (2) year period beginning on the date the affidavit is signed. A copy of the affidavit must be filed with the Secretary of HHS within ten (10) days after the first **private contract** to which the affidavit applies is entered into.

Should a physician or practitioner in signing the affidavit knowingly and willfully submit a Medicare claim, or receive Medicare reimbursement, for an item or service during such two (2) year period, the ability to provide services under the **private contract** will cease for the remainder of the period. Further, the physician or practitioner may not receive any Medicare payments during such period.

APPENDIX H

COORDINATION OF COVERAGE – MEDICARE AND EMPLOYER PLANS

The several types of **coordination of Medicare and employer plans** coverage are set forth below:

I. CARVE-OUT COVERAGE.

The plan deducts the amount that Medicare pays for services from a scheduled amount set forth in the plan representing a charge for the same services, and the plan pays the difference.

II. WRAP-AROUND COVERAGE.

This is somewhat like **Medigap** insurance and will typically cover Medicare cost-sharing requirements and supplemental benefits, such as **prescription drugs**, **preventive care** and **dental care**.

III. COORDINATION OF BENEFITS COVERAGE.

The plan in most cases will pay the difference between the actual charge and the **Medicare-allowed charge** up to an amount scheduled in the plan. The effect of this coverage is that Medicare will pay for Medicare-covered services, and to the extent that Medicare does not cover, the services will be subject to the plan's coinsurance requirements.

IV. EXCLUSION COVERAGE.

Medicare payments are subtracted from the **actual charge** for services, and the plan will pay the balance subject to the beneficiary's responsibility for the plan's cost-sharing and deductible provisions.

CHAPTER 4

MEDICAID
A FEDERAL AND STATE SOURCE OF PAYMENT

Introduction

Medicaid (Title XIX of the Social Security Act) is a **welfare program of medical assistance**. Financed jointly by the state and Federal governments, the program is administered by each state separately. Each state operates its own Medicaid program under rules established by the Federal government and state-specific laws and regulations.

Medicaid is a means-tested program. Unlike Medicare (which is available regardless of financial need to most persons **age 65 or older** and to certain disabled individuals), Medicaid is **available only to individuals with limited income and resources.** All the states plus Puerto Rico, the Virgin Islands, Guam and the District of Columbia participate in Medicaid; Arizona has a limited program. Within the Medicaid program, there are several sub-programs known as **Buy-in Programs** or **Medical Savings Programs**. They assist low-income Medicaid beneficiaries to pay some or all of the **premiums, co-payments** and **deductibles** associated with the Medicaid program. There are several categories of low-income individuals – namely, Qualified Medicare Beneficiaries, Specified Low-income Medicare Beneficiaries, and Qualifying Individuals. These beneficiaries may "buy-in" to the sub-programs without applying for full Medicaid coverage. The payments are made by state Medicaid agencies.

At the Federal level, the **Department of Health and Human Services (HHS)**, through the **Centers of Medicare and Medicaid Services (CMS)**, issues regulations and guidelines and monitors state compliance with Federal laws and rules. HHS publishes the *State Medical Assistance Manual* for use by the states in administering the program. **At the state level**, a state agency is responsible for issuing rules and regulations and guidelines for Medicaid eligibility. **Local agencies** are responsible for day-to-day administration of the Medicaid program.

The Medicaid program enables a Medicaid recipient to receive medical services. The bill of the Medicaid individual for medical services received is sent to the state Medicaid agency for payment. Each Medicaid recipient gets a **plastic identification card,** which must be presented when services are received. Medicaid pays doctors, hospitals, nursing homes and other providers directly, provided they have agreed to accept Medicaid clients and agree to accept Medicaid payment as payment in full.

Individuals age 65 and over, blind or disabled persons, low-income pregnant women and certain low-income families with children may qualify for Medicaid assistance. Medicaid recipients must be **American citizens** or fall within specified categories of **permanent resident aliens**.

In general, states serve two groups of persons through their Medicaid programs. First, states must serve the **categorically needy,** defined to include aged (65 years and older), blind, and disabled persons eligible for benefits under the Supplemental Security Income (SSI) program. Second, states are permitted, but not required, to serve the **medically needy**, which refers to those persons in need of medical assistance whose income levels disqualify them from the SSI program.

Congress created the SSI program in 1972, to take effect January 1, 1974. The new SSI eligibility criteria were broader than some of the prior state-established criteria. Congress added **§209(b) to the Supplemental Security Income Act**, 42 U.S.C. § 1396a(f), to encourage continued participation by states with stricter criteria. States choosing the **§ 209(b) option** are not required to provide Medicaid to persons who would not have been eligible under the state medical assistance plan in effect on January 1, 1972, prior to the enactment of SSI. The 209(b) states are: Connecticut, Hawaii, Illinois, Indiana, Minnesota, Missouri, Nebraska, New Hampshire, North Carolina, North Dakota, Ohio, Oklahoma, Utah and Virginia.

States electing the 209(b) option are required (with few exceptions) to operate a program for the medical needy and to adopt a spend-down process.

When a "medically needy" applicant's income or resources exceed the applicable state's Medicaid eligibility limits, the "spend down" process may apply. Under this process, the applicant may be able to "spend down" excess income or resources, by applying them to outstanding medical bills, to become eligible for Medicaid. **Income spend-down** is the process whereby an applicant's income is reduced for the purpose of determining Medicaid eligibility by the amount of incurred but unpaid medical expenses. **Resource spend-down** is the process which allows Medicaid applicants to offset their resources by incurred but unpaid medical bills.

The Balanced Budget Act of 1997 amended the Social Security Act so that **states may require individuals eligible for Medicaid medical assistance to enroll in a managed care entity.**

This chapter will outline broad Medicaid rules in reference to:

Chapter 4 | Introduction to Medicaid
(continued)

- **ELIGIBILITY REQUIREMENTS** (see section I below);
- **TRANSFER OF ASSETS PENALTY RULES** (see section II below);
- **MEDICAID HOME CARE BENEFITS** (see section III below);
- **MEDICAID APPEALS** (see section IV below);
- **MANDATORY MANAGED CARE** (see section V below); and
- **STATE LONG-TERM PARTNERSHIP PROGRAMS** (see section VI below).

Chapter 4   Eligibility

I. WHAT ARE THE ELIGIBILITY CRITERIA FOR MEDICAID?

A. What Are the Factors to Establish Medicaid Eligibility?

There are several factors that determine whether an applicant is eligible for Medicaid or not.

- An applicant has to be a **U.S. citizen** or fall within specified categories of **permanent resident aliens**;
- Status Standards (see B below);
- Income Standards (see C below);
- Resource Standards (see D below);
- Married Couple Income and Resource Standards (see E below);
- Categories of Medicaid-eligibles (see F below);
- Trust Eligibility Rules (see G below);
- State Optional Standards (see H below).

B. What Are the Status Standards?

The applicant must be <u>elderly (age 65 and over)</u> with <u>limited income and resources</u>, or disabled or blind (at any age) with limited income and resources. Some other categories of potentially eligible persons include: low-income pregnant women, and some low-income families with children. Some states consider all people eligible for Supplemental Security Income assistance to be automatically eligible for Medicaid.

C. What Are the Income Standards?

An applicant has to have **countable income** that is $725/month (2008) for an individual and $1,067/month (2008) for a couple (these figures may differ in some states). Some states allow people with higher incomes to **spend down** (see section I.F(2)) a portion of their income on needed health care in order to become eligible for Medicaid coverage of any remaining health care costs.

1. <u>What Is Considered Countable Income for Medicaid Purposes?</u>

The term "countable income" means any recurring payment from any source and of any kind (money, goods or services). It includes one-half of monthly **earned income** (such as a salary or self-employment); **unearned**

income (such as a pension, Social Security benefits or investment profits); and **in-kind income** (such as food, clothing, or shelter obtained from another person). All sources of income are combined to determine the applicant's so-called countable income that will determine whether the applicant is eligible for Medicaid or not. To be counted, the income must be **available** to the Medicaid applicant; that is, within his/her possession or control or obtained with reasonable effort.

The **available income** of married couples is pooled together in calculating the financial eligibility of the applicant spouse as if the total income were that of the applicant (see section I.E below).

D. What Are the Resource Standards?

An applicant has to meet the resource limitations that are determined in each state. Allowable resources, such as savings, cannot be more than $4,350(individual)/$6,400(couple). States have rules that prohibit transferring assets for the sole purpose of becoming eligible for Medicaid.

1. What Are Considered Countable Resources for Medicaid Programs?

The term "countable resource" includes cash on hand; stocks and bonds; certificates of deposit; mutual fund shares; bank accounts (including joint accounts); pension funds; retirement funds; insurance; real property (other than **homestead** (see D.2 below)); and entrance fees for a continuing care retirement community.

To be counted the resource must be "available" to the Medicaid applicant. Assets that belong to the applicant's spouse or that are owned jointly are considered available to the applicant and will also be counted as an "available resource."

2. Does Medicaid Allow Any Resource Exemptions?

Yes. Certain resources are not counted by Medicaid in determining an individual's eligibility for benefits. States must exempt the following resources:

- a **home** (not exceeding $500,000 in value and in some states $750,000) so long as the person lives there (or intends to return there), or as long as a spouse or disabled or dependent children live there;

- household goods and personal effects;
- an automobile;
- a burial space (or the value of an agreement to purchase a burial space);
- a separate bank account set aside for burial expenses of no more than $1,500;
- life insurance policies with a face value of $1,500 or less, regardless of surrender value. The combined value of the burial fund and the face value of a life insurance policy may not exceed $1,500 in the aggregate; and
- up to $6,000 equity in non-business property (personal or real estate) that produces net annual income of at least six (6) percent of the amount of the protected property (for example, farm equipment needed to grow food for an individual's own consumption).

E. **Are the Income and Resource Eligibility Standards Which Apply to Single Individuals Applicable to Married Couples?**

No.

The standards, as set forth below, are different.

1. **Deeming of Income and Resources of Spouses. Medicaid rules impose upon married couples the financial responsibility to provide for one another.** The Medicaid applicant's available income and non-exempt income resources, and the available income and non-exempt resources of the other spouse are pooled together and counted as available to the other spouse in calculating the applicant's financial eligibility for Medicaid. This is known as the **Rule of Deeming** (see section E.2 below).

   When one spouse is institutionalized and applies for Medicaid, that individual (**Applicant Spouse**) is known as the **Institutionalized Spouse**. The person who is married to the institutionalized spouse and who remains in the community is known as the **Community Spouse**. Applying the Rule of Deeming mentioned above, the income (earned and unearned) and resources (excluding those exempted) of the community

Chapter 4

Eligibility
(continued)

spouse who is not applying for Medicaid are "deemed" available to, and added to those of, the applicant institutionalized spouse.

Medicaid will make an assessment of resources of a couple (the colloquial term "**snapshot rule**" refers to the act of assessing), for the purposes of Medicaid eligibility, at the beginning of a period of institutionalization of one member of the couple. A snapshot of the couple's resources is taken when one begins a nursing home stay expected to last a period of thirty (30) days or more (**continuous period of institutionalization**), regardless of whether an application is made at that time (see sections E.3-4). The non-exempt resources of the couple are pooled as of the snapshot day.

2. **When Deeming Ceases**

    Deeming ceases upon the occurrence of the following events:

    - **When a married couple stops living together other than for reason of institutionalization** (e.g., divorce), the couple's income and resources are counted as available to each other for the month the couple ceases living together, and for the ensuing six- (6) month period. Thereafter, deeming ceases, and each of the previously married spouses is treated as a single individual.

    - **When a married couple stops living together upon institutionalization of one of them**.

    - **Deeming will also cease** when one spouse (applicant) who resides in the community and needs Medicaid community service and home care services all of which are **non-waivered services**, and the non-applicant spouse submits a written letter to Medicaid (**Spousal Refusal Letter**) that he/she is unable to unwilling to contribute financial support to the applicant spouse (see section E.5). Once the letter is submitted to Medicaid, along with the applicant's **Medicaid application**, the applicant will be considered as a single individual by Medicaid. Medicaid will thus base its eligibility determination for the non-waivered services solely on the income and resources of the applicant.

Chapter 4   **Eligibility**
                                                                                                                        (continued)

3. **Protection of Community Spouse Against Impoverishment**

    Medicaid restricts the amount of income and assets a Medicaid applicant is allowed to retain after **institutionalization**. This could lead to the impoverishment of the community spouse. Consequently, states are required to permit an institutionalized individual (or at states' option, an individual who is a recipient of waivered home health benefits), who is married and receives Medicaid assistance, to contribute to his/her spouse, remaining in the community in order to bring that community spouse's <u>income</u>, up to a **Minimum Monthly Income Allowance** and <u>resources</u> up to a **Minimum Resource Allowance**. In addition, the community spouse is assured a **Family Allowance** (for family dependents living with the community spouse) and an **Excess Shelter Allowance**.

    <u>Medicaid will make an assessment of resources of a couple</u>, at the request of either the community spouse or the applicant, and may do so at any time of the institutionalization of the applicant. The colloquial term "**snapshot rule**" refers to the act of assessing, for the purposes of Medicaid eligibility, at the beginning of a period of institutionalization of one member of the couple. A snapshot of the couple's resources is taken when one begins a nursing home stay expected to last a period of thirty (30) days or more (**continuous period of institutionalization**), regardless of whether an **application** is made at that time. **The non-exempt resources of the couple are pooled as of the snapshot day.** <u>Following the assessment</u>, Medicaid will determine the Medicaid eligibility amount for the community spouse minimum monthly income allowance, **excess shelter allowance**, and family allowance <u>based on the following factors</u>:

    - States are required to adopt <u>the Community Spouse Minimum Monthly Income Allowance</u> (**Basic Allowance**) for the community spouse which is equal to one-hundred fifty (150) percent of the then Federal poverty level for a two- (2) person family (even though the community spouse is only one person). This amounts to a minimum monthly gross allowance of $1,750 (2008). The allowance is adjusted annually for inflation.

Chapter 4	Eligibility
	(continued)

- States are also required to calculate and provide an <u>excess shelter allowance</u> where the costs (e.g., rent, mortgage, taxes, maintenance charges on a co-op, insurance and utilities) of maintaining the principal residence exceeds thirty (30) percent of the applicable percentage of the poverty level. The **excess shelter allowance** will be added to the basic allowance.

- In addition, states are required to provide a **family allowance** (see section E.7) below).

- There is a cap of $2,610 (2008) as adjusted by inflation, on the total of the basic allowance and the excess shelter allowance.

- In lieu of the allowance computed with the above two components (basic allowance and excess shelter allowance) a state may elect a **flat monthly maintenance allowance**. (California and New York have, for example, made this election.) This allowance is subject to a cap of $2,610 (2008) indexed for inflation.

- The amount allowed for the community spouse, whether consisting of the basic allowance plus excess shelter allowance, or the flat monthly allowance, <u>may be increased</u> at a Fair Hearing on the grounds of "exceptional circumstances resulting in significant financial duress requiring the provision of additional income."

- <u>If the community spouse resource allowance is insufficient</u> to generate the statutory Minimum Monthly Income Allowance, the community spouse <u>may resort to a Fair Hearing</u> to increase his/her resource allowance to make up the income deficiency. However, the community spouse <u>may not resort to the Fair Hearing process</u> to increase his/her <u>resource allowance</u> unless the institutionalized spouse has first made available to the community spouse, out of his/her income, an amount sufficient to make up the deficiency. (This is referred to as the **Income First Rule**).

4. <u>**Spousal Share – Maximum and Minimum Community Spouse Resource Allowance**</u>.

   In determining the eligibility of an institutionalized person with a spouse in the community, Medicaid provides that the community spouse must be allowed to **retain** resources (**spousal share**) equal to one-half of the couple's assessed total countable resources, but not less than the **minimum community spouse resource allowance**, and not more than the **maximum community spouse resource allowance** permitted under Federal law – $20,880 (2008) and $104,400 (2008), respectively.

The spousal share is determined by the spouse as of the beginning of the most recent continuous period of institutionalization of the institutionalized spouse. **Continuous period of institutionalization** means at least thirty (30) consecutive days of institutional care in a medical institution and/or nursing facility, or receipt of home and community-based waiver services, or a combination of institutional and home and community-based waiver services.

5. **Spousal Refusal – When the Community Spouse's Spousal Share Exceeds the Community Spouse Maximum Resource Allowance.**

    As noted above, the minimum community spouse resource allowance is $20,880 (2008), and the maximum community spouse resource allowance is $104,400 (2008). If the spousal share (i.e., one-half of the combined countable resources of both spouses) exceeds $20,880 (2008), the community spouse is allowed to retain resources in an amount equal to the spousal share but not to exceed $104,400 (2008). **If, in fact, the community spouse has resources in excess of the spousal share, the excess is considered to be available to the institutionalized spouse**, and the community spouse is required to contribute the excess amount to the cost of care of the institutionalized spouse. If the community spouse should fail or refuse to contribute these excess resources, the refusal is termed "Spousal Refusal." In cases of a spousal refusal, the resources of the community spouse will no longer be considered available to the institutionalized spouse. However, the latter can still receive Medicaid:

    – if the institutionalized spouse assigned to the state rights to support from the community spouse;

    – if the institutionalized spouse lacks the ability to execute an assignment due to physical or mental impairment, but the state has the right to bring a support proceeding against the community spouse; or

Chapter 4

Eligibility
(continued)

      – if denial of eligibility would work an undue hardship.

6. **When the Community Spouse's Spousal Share Is Less than the Minimum Community Spouse Resource Allowance.**

   The institutionalized spouse is required to transfer to the community spouse an amount sufficient to increase the latter's resources up to the spousal share. This transfer to the sole name of the community spouse should be made within ninety (90) days of the initial eligibility determination in order to protect the spousal allowance from consideration as an available resource of the institutionalized spouse. Resources not shifted by the deadline will be considered available resources of the institutionalized spouse.

7. **Permitted Deductions.**

   The Medicaid statute is designed to require application of all of the income of the institutionalized spouse, <u>after</u> **permitted deductions**, to the cost of institutional care. These permitted deductions (including the institutionalized spouse's **personal needs allowance** (PNA)) are set forth below:

   - The <u>community spouse's monthly income allowance</u>;
   - <u>Personal needs allowance</u> (see 8 below);
   - <u>A family allowance</u> for each family member (who is residing with the community spouse and who has over fifty (50) percent of his/her maintenance needs met by the community spouse and/or the institutionalized spouse – an amount equal to at least one-third of the amount by which the minimum monthly needs allowance (not including the excess shelter allowance) exceeds the amount of the monthly income of that family member.
   - Amounts for incurred <u>expenses for medical or remedial care for the institutionalized spouse</u>.
   - States may deduct an <u>amount for the maintenance of the home</u> of the institutionalized spouse for six (6) months or less if a physician certifies that the individual is likely to return home within that period.

8. **Personal Needs Allowance.**

   This is an amount of money required to be set aside for an **institutionalized individual receiving nursing facility services** in

Long-term Care at Home Consumer Guide

order to pay for personal needs such as clothing, reading material, stationery, and snacks not required to be provided by the facility, and activities not required to be provided by the facility. **At a minimum, the allowance must be $50 per month. States can increase the PNA above the minimum.**

The PNA also applies (except as to amount) to **institutionalized spouses living in the community and either receiving a waiver service or participating in the Program of All-inclusive Care for the Elderly (PACE).** The PNA amount for such persons is higher than the $50 PNA that institutionalized residents are allowed to retain. The PNA amount for institutionalized spouses living in the community and receiving waiver services or participating in PACE is $342/month, effective January 1, 2008.

F.   **What Are the Categories of Eligibility?**

There are three significant categories of SSI and Medicaid-eligibles: categorically needy, optional categorically needy, and medically needy. (Also, there are miscellaneous categories of eligibility set forth in (4) below.)

1. **Categorically Needy.**

    All states must provide Medicaid coverage to persons who are in the categorically needy group. This is one of the three main groups of potential Medicaid-eligible persons (i.e., categorically needy, optional categorically needy and medically needy). An individual, otherwise eligible for Medicaid, who satisfies the SSI financial eligibility standards of a state's Medicaid program, historically is considered to be eligible for Medicaid as categorically needy. More specifically, the classification describes individuals who satisfy the categorical requirements of being age 65 or over or being blind or disabled, and in addition satisfy a state's Medicaid financial eligibility requirements of having assets or income below state-determined levels.

    In most states an individual who receives SSI is automatically considered to be within this group. **A person who is categorically needy is not allowed to spend down.**

Chapter 4

Eligibility
(continued)

2. **Medically Needy.**

   The **medically needy** group is optional to states. Thirty-seven (37) states and the District of Columbia have this category. It is for persons who meet the non-financial status requirements (age, disability) for categorical assistance, but whose income and/or resources are over the categorical needy levels. Unlike the categorically needy or optional categorically needy, **a medically needy person has the right to reduce his/her income to below state-prescribed levels through the deduction of incurred medical expenses, a process referred to above as "spending down."**

   The medically needy programs will not necessarily provide to a "spendowner" all requisite medical assistance. A state with a medically needy program may elect to provide nursing home facilities or not. In those states whose programs do provide nursing home facilities to the medically needy, the expenses which may be deducted from countable income and resources are both the individual's medical and nursing home expenses. In those states whose programs do not provide nursing home facilities, individuals cannot spend down to become nursing home eligible – i.e., there is no spend down for the incurred or paid medical expenses in order to obtain eligibility for nursing home care.

3. **Optional Categorically Needy.**

   States that do not have a medically needy program serving nursing facility residents are referred to an "income cap" states. In these states individuals **are not allowed to spend down to the SSI income level** to become eligible for Medicaid-covered nursing home care. **These states (income cap states) avail themselves of an optional Medicaid program termed the optional categorically needy program under which individuals are provided limited nursing facility coverage.** Under the program individuals qualify for Medicaid nursing home coverage if their countable income does not exceed a cap of a prescribed percentage, usually three-hundred (300) percent, of the SSI benefit for one person. The three-hundred (300)

<u>percent cap is an absolute dollar cap</u>. It is categorically fixed and severe: one dollar of excess income above the cap will disqualify the individual. **An individual is not permitted to spend down for medical expenses, nor can he/she forego collection of a pension, Social Security benefits or interest income in order to fall within the income cap.** <u>The income cap states are Alabama, Alaska, Colorado, Delaware, Idaho, Mississippi, Nevada, New Mexico, Ohio, South Dakota and Wyoming</u>.

A possible method for reducing the income of an individual seeking to qualify under the optional categorically needy program, also <u>commonly referred to as the three-hundred (300) percent program</u>, is to obtain from a state court a qualified domestic relations order which allocates pension payments to the community spouse. The community spouse as the payee arguably is the beneficiary of the pension, and payments to him/her would constitute his/her income under the name-on-the-check rule, not income of the institutionalized spouse who was the original pensioner.

Another method of qualifying for the optional categorically needy program is available under the provisions of the Consolidated Omnibus Budget Reconciliation Act of 1993. With this law **Congress allowed individuals in income cap states to become eligible for Medicaid nursing home assistance by putting their income (e.g., pension, Social Security benefits) into a so-called Miller trust**. During the Medicaid recipient's lifetime, all but a small portion of the money in the trust must go toward paying the nursing home bill. If any money remains in the trust after the recipient's death, it must be paid to the state, up to the amount of Medicaid assistance that was rendered.

Chapter 4	Eligibility
	(continued)

4. **Low-income Medicare Beneficiaries.** Medicaid will pay certain Medicare benefits (deductibles, co-payments, coinsurance, and/or premiums) for low-income Medicare beneficiaries, as set forth below:

a) Qualified Medicare Beneficiary (QMB). Federal law requires state Medicaid programs to **buy-in Medicare coverage** for certain low-income Medicare beneficiaries. The buy-in consists of payment of deductibles and coinsurance costs under Medicare Part A and Part B, payment of premiums under Part B, and payment of premiums under Part A for those not entitled to Part A by virtue of receiving Social Security benefits. These beneficiaries are known as Qualified Medicare Beneficiaries (QMB).

QMBs must:

- meet federally prescribed income and resource standards. Individuals must have incomes below one-hundred (100) percent of the **Federal poverty level**, and their non-exempt resources cannot exceed twice the SSI resource standard ($4,000 for an individual and $6,000 for a family of two).

- be entitled to Part A hospital insurance. If they otherwise would be eligible for QMB benefits but are not automatically eligible for Medicare Part A, the state must pay their Part A premiums to make them eligible for Part A.

[A subset of QMBs is known as **Dual Eligibles**. They are individuals who have low assets and are eligible for full coverage under both Medicare and Medicaid. They are exempt from mandatory enrollment in Medicaid managed care. Virtually all individuals receiving Medicaid or age 65 and over are entitled to Medicare Part B at least. A state's Medicaid program pays the Medicare Part B premiums for dual eligibles and should also pay Medicare Part A premiums for those not entitled to Part A by virtue of receiving Social Security retirement benefits. All dual eligibles are Qualified Medicare

Chapter 4   **Eligibility**
                                                                                                                            (continued)

Beneficiaries, but not all QMBs are duly eligible. They are entitled to the full spectrum of both Medicaid and Medicare benefits.]

b) <u>Specified Low-income Medicare Beneficiary (SLMB)</u>. An individual entitled to Medicare Part A benefits whose income is between one-hundred (100) percent and one-hundred twenty (120) percent of Federal poverty guidelines and whose non-exempt resources are $4,000 or less ($6,000 in the case of a couple) is eligible to have Medicaid pay his/her Medicare Part B premium. This individual is referred to as a SLMB with the Qualified Medicare Beneficiary program. The SLMB program is managed by the state agency that provides medical assistance under Medicaid.

c) <u>Low-income Qualifying Individual (QI-1)</u>. An individual is selected by the state as a qualifying individual (QI-1). A QI-1 must meet the QMB criteria, except that his/her income level is at least one-hundred twenty (120) percent but less than one-hundred thirty-five (135) percent of the Federal poverty level for a family of the size involved and his/her non-exempt resources are $4,000 or less ($6,000 in the case of a couple). There is no asset test in New York and some other states. The state is required to pay the full amount of the Medicare Part B premiums of such a qualifying individual (but only the premiums payable during a statutorily prescribed period). However, a QI-1 cannot be otherwise eligible for medical assistance under the approved state Medicaid plan.

d) <u>Qualified Disabled and Working Individuals (QDWI)</u>. State Medicaid programs must pay Medicare Part A premiums for the individuals whose income is below two-hundred (200) percent of the Federal poverty level; who are entitled to Medicare on the basis of disability; who are in a trial work period and are entitled to continue Medicare coverage while they are in that work period; whose resources do not exceed twice SSI resource levels ($4,000 for individuals plus $1,500 for burial expenses, and $6,000 plus $3,000 for burial expenses in the case of couples); and who are not otherwise eligible for Medicaid.

G. **According to Medicaid Trust Eligibility Rules, Is the Principal or the Income of Trusts Created by the Applicant Considered Countable Resources or Countable Income?**

It depends:

1. <u>If the trust is a living (*inter vivos*) revocable trust (as defined below)</u>, the income and principal are considered to be countable and may affect the Medicaid eligibility.

   A living (*inter vivos*) revocable trust is created by a grantor during his/her lifetime and may be amended or revoked by the grantor at any time or at the end of a designated period. The trust may be funded at the time of the trust's creation by the transfer of assets to it, or left unfunded until the occurrence of some event.

2. <u>If the trust is a testamentary trust, neither the principal nor the income is considered to be countable</u> and thus does not affect the applicant's Medicaid eligibility.

   A testamentary trust is created by the last will and testament of the grantor (the testator) and becomes effective after the testator's death. If the testamentary trust is created by a community spouse for the benefit of his/her surviving spouse who is institutionalized, to avoid the principal or income from being countable and available to the institutionalized spouse (and thereby affecting his/her Medicaid eligibility), the trust must contain provisions which prevent, under any circumstances, the distribution of the trust principal to the institutionalized spouse, and may permit the payment of the trust income for the comfort and happiness of the institutionalized spouse, but not for food, clothing or shelter.

3. <u>If the trust is a life time (*inter vivos*) irrevocable trust</u>, under the terms of which applicant loses all control over the trust asset (principal), and the asset and income are transferred to another

Chapter 4   **Eligibility**
(continued)

beneficiary, <u>neither the principal nor the income is countable</u> so that the applicant's Medicaid eligibility is not affected.

An irrevocable living trust is created by a grantor during his/her lifetime for purposes of irrevocably transferring assets to another beneficiary. The grantor loses all control over the trust assets (principal) and may not amend or revoke the trust.

4. <u>Applicability of Trust Rules to Supplemental Needs Trust</u> – This type of trust, also known as a **special needs trust**, is an irrevocable trust, funded by assets of a third party, created for a disabled beneficiary, and intended to supplement government benefits. The trust prohibits the trustee from spending trust assets in diminution of government benefits. The beneficiary has no power to control distributions. Generally, for Medicaid eligibility purposes, payments from a **supplemental needs trust** are governed by SSI income principles. If payments are made for food, clothing or shelter, or if payments are made directly to the beneficiary, the amounts are counted as income to the beneficiary for purposes of eligibility and will disqualify the beneficiary's Medicaid eligibility status. <u>The more common arrangement with supplemental needs trusts, which will not disqualify the beneficiary's Medicaid eligibility, is for the trustee to make direct payments to vendors of services or goods that are not food, clothing or shelter</u>, such payments are not considered income to the beneficiary.

5. <u>Exempt Trusts</u> – Three categories of established trusts are by statute expressly considered exempt from the Medicaid trust eligibility rules. One trust (**income-only trust**) is exempt by virtue of an administrative ruling.

   (a) **Trust for Disabled Person under Age 65**. This trust contains the disabled person's assets and is established for his/her benefit by his/her parent, grandparent, legal guardian or a court. This trust is exempt from the Medicaid eligibility rules if it provides that the state will receive all amounts remaining in the trust upon the death of the disabled person up to the amount of Medicaid assistance provided to this person by the state.

(b) **Miller Trust**. This trust is composed of an individual's pension or Social Security income and is exempt from Medicaid eligibility rules if the following conditions are met:

- The trust is composed only of the individual's pension, Social Security, or other income payable to the individual, including accumulated trust income. Neither the income transferred to this type of trust nor the right to recover the income is counted in determining the individual's eligibility for Medicaid.

- The state will receive all amounts remaining in the trust upon the person's death up to the amount of Medicaid assistance provided to this person by the state.

- The individual resides in a state, commonly known as an income cap state or "300%" state, that does not have a medically needy program for nursing facility services and that uses a special income limit for eligibility for certain long-term care services.

Should any principal be transferred to a Miller trust, this will disqualify the trust from its exempt status. A transfer to the trust of the ownership rights to a stream of income (e.g., Social Security benefits) constitutes a transfer of a resource and will also cause the trust to lose its exempt status.

(c) **Pooled Trust**. This trust is established for a disabled individual, regardless of age, and contains the assets of that individual. If it meets certain conditions, a pooled trust is exempt from Medicaid eligibility rules:

- The trust is established and managed by a nonprofit association.

- Each trust beneficiary has a separate account, but the trust pools these accounts for investment and management of the funds.

- These accounts are established solely for the disabled individual's benefit by the individual, the individual's parent, grandparent, or legal guardian, or by a court.

- Any amounts remaining in the trust after the beneficiary's death and not retained by it are paid over to

Chapter 4   **Eligibility**
                                                                           (continued)

the state up to an amount equal to the total amount of Medicaid services provided to the beneficiary.

(d) **Income-only Trust**. This trust is an *inter vivos* irrevocable trust established by an individual. It provides that only income shall be paid to the grantor for life, but excludes distribution of principal to the grantor. CMS has interpreted the Medicaid eligibility trust rules to preclude the counting of such trust's principal as available to the grantor since it cannot under any circumstances be distributed to, or for the benefit of, the grantor or his/her spouse.

H. What Are Some Other State Eligibility Standards?

1. In most but not all states, individuals who satisfy the eligibility conditions for the Federal Supplemental Security Income (SSI) program (a program for the indigent elderly, blind, or disabled), are **automatically eligible** for Medicaid in addition to being eligible for SSI.

2. Some states cover people who are not eligible for SSI because their income is higher than the SSI income limits. In these states people who are close to the eligibility limit are permitted to reduce their net income to the Medicaid income limits by deducting from their income all incurred medical care expenses. Thus, by paying privately for some medical expenses, they are spending down to the Medicaid income limit; once they have done so, Medicaid will cover any additional medical cost they may have. This is a particularly important provision for people who have high monthly medical expenses, but it is not available in all states.

3. Some states have elected to provide Medicaid coverage for nursing home care only for people whose gross income does not exceed three-hundred (300) percent of the SSI benefit rate in that state. These states (**income cap states**) may set the eligibility level anywhere between the SSI rate and three-hundred (300) percent of that rate. The three-hundred (300) percent cap, however, is an absolute dollar cap, and an individual whose gross income is above this cap cannot spend down, the way this can be done in other states.

Chapter 4   *Transfer of Assets Penalty Rules*

II. WHAT ARE THE PENALTY RULES FOR THE TRANSFER OF ASSETS?

A. Can One Transfer Assets or Property to Become Medicaid Eligible?

Generally no.

As a general rule, anyone who is elderly or disabled, and who is considering the need for home care or nursing home care now or in the future, should not during the individual's life, transfer any money or goods during a prescribed period of months (**look-back period**) immediately prior to applying for Medicaid. Historically, this period was 36 months for all transfers, except that transfers into a trust were subject to a 60-month look-back period; the 36-month period has been extended to 60 months (as a prescribed basis) so that the look-back period for all transfers (other than to or from **Exempt Trusts**) will be a 60-month period (See Phase-in Table on next page). Such a transfer of assets may cause the applicant, who may otherwise be eligible for Medicaid, to be found ineligible for a period of time (**period of ineligibility**).

B. What Is a Look-back Period?

As described above, the term "look-back period" refers to a number of months prior to the Medicaid application for which the Medicaid agency will ask the applicant to account for any transfers of assets, including transfers for less than fair market value. States must use the federally designated look-back period.

The commencement date of the look-back period in the case of an institutionalized person is the date the individual is deemed both an institutionalized person and an applicant for state Medicaid assistance. In the case of a non-institutionalized person, the commencement date is the date that the individual applies for state Medicaid aid, or, if later, the date that the individual disposes of assets for less than fair market value.

- In the case of transfer of assets made before the date of enactment (the "enactment date") of the Deficit Reduction Act of 2005 (DRA), the commencement date is the first day of the first month during or after the assets have been transferred for less than fair market value and which does not occur during any other period of ineligibility.

Chapter 4

Transfer of Assets Penalty Rules
(continued)

- In the case of transfer of assets made <u>on or after</u> the enactment date of the DRA, the commencement date is (i) the first day of the month during or after which assets have been transferred for less than fair market value <u>or</u> (ii) the date on which the individual is eligible for medical assistance under the state plan <u>and</u> would otherwise be receiving institutional level care (e.g., nursing home facility services), but for the application of the penalty period, **whichever is later** and which does not occur during any other period of ineligibility.

<u>When multiple transfers are made</u> during the look-back period, they are treated as follows:

- For multiple transfers during the look-back period when assets have been transferred in amounts or in frequency that would make the calculated periods overlap, the transfers must be added together and then divided by the average monthly payment for nursing facilities within a state, or, at the option of the state, within a designated region of the state. <u>The total amount transferred will be treated as if it was all transferred over on the first day of the month following the month in which the first transfer is made</u>.

- When multiple transfers are made in such a way that the penalties for each do not even overlap, <u>each transfer is treated as a separate event, with its own penalty period</u>.

Phase-in of Extended Look-back Period

Phase-in Period	Extension of Look-back Period
1993 until Jan. 30, 2009	36 months
February 1, 2009	36 + 1 = 37 months
March 1, 2009	36 + 2 = 38 months
Every month through Feb. 1, 2011	Look-back period extended by 1 month
February 1, 2010	36 + 13 = 49 months
February 1, 2011	60 months

Chapter 4   **Transfer of Assets Penalty Rules**
                                                                                 (continued)

C.   What Is a Prohibited Transfer of Assets?

Certain gifts or transactions that were made during a **prescribed period (look-back period)** prior to an individual's submission of a Medicaid application, will be considered prohibited transfers of assets <u>for less than fair market value</u>, and will result in a **period of ineligibility** (the **transfer penalty**) for the person who made the transfer. The penalty is imposed **when a person <u>transfers any asset</u> for less than fair market value** (called **uncompensated value** of transferred assets), and applies for Medicaid assistance to pay for certain long-term care services **during the look-back period**.

The term "assets," as used in the context of the Medicaid transfer of assets penalty rule, includes:

- the income and resources of a Medicaid applicant/recipient or such individual's spouse which either have been placed in a trust <u>or</u> have been transferred to someone else for less than fair market value.

- an annuity purchased by the Medicaid applicant/recipient is considered as the transfer of an asset for less than fair market value <u>unless</u> the annuity meets specific requirements:

    i) The state is either the remainder beneficiary in the first position for at least the full amount of medical assistance received by the Medicaid recipient; or

    ii) The state is listed as the beneficiary in the second position after the community spouse of disabled or minor child; and the state is named in the first position if either the spouse or the child's representative disposes of the remainder of the annuity for less than fair market value.

- funds of the Medicaid applicant/recipient used to purchase a mortgage, or for a loan or promissory note unless the repayment terms is actuarially sound, provides for payments in equal amounts during the term of the loan without deferrals or balloon payments, and prohibits the cancellation on the lender's death.

- income or resources which a Medicaid applicant/recipient is entitled to but does not receive because of his/her own actions, such as a disclaimer, waiver of pension income, or waiver of his inheritance.

Prohibited transfers include:

- gifts;
- funds exchanged for an item for less than its fair market value;
- significant withdrawals of funds from a checking or savings account that cannot be documented as purchases for fair market value; and
- transfers to create certain kinds of exempt trusts. (The creation of some trusts (**exempt trusts**) will not affect Medicaid eligibility.)

The transfer penalty must be applied in cases of individuals seeking nursing home care, or its equivalent, and/or waivered home care services. It affects Medicaid non-waivered home care services, only if a state so elects.

D. What Is the Penalty for Making a Prohibited Transfer of Assets?

When a transfer of assets has taken place, the Medicaid program will presume that the transfer of assets was made for the purpose of becoming Medicaid-eligible for certain Medicaid services. This presumption can be overcome, if the applicant can demonstrate (with the proper documentation) that the transfer was made for another purpose. The penalty for a prohibited transfer of assets in most cases will be that the applicant will **not** be eligible for Medicaid for a certain period of time (**period of ineligibility**).

E. What Is the Period of Ineligibility?

This period is a number of months that an individual has made a transfer of assets for less than fair market value within the look-back period. During this period an individual shall remain ineligible for designated services. For an institutionalized person, the period of ineligibility equals, and for a non-institutionalized person is not greater than, the number of months calculated by dividing: (i) the total uncompensated value of all assets an individual disposed of during the look-back period by (ii) a patient's average cost of nursing facility care per month.

Chapter 4 **Transfer of Assets Penalty Rules**
(continued)

It is emphasized that the penalty consists of the imposition of the period of ineligibility for Medicaid assistance covering **only** certain **designated services** as defined in section H below.

F.   Are Any Transfers Not Subject to a Penalty?

Yes. Certain transfers of assets are **exempt** from the penalty rules and will not trigger a penalty. These include:

- transfers for fair market value (purchasing an item or service for fair market value, even if it is a luxury item);

- transfers made exclusively for a purpose other than becoming Medicaid-eligible (detailed documentation will be required to overcome Medicaid's presumption that the transfer was made for Medicaid purposes);

- transfers to or from an individual's spouse;

- transfers to a child under age 21 or to a disabled child (of any age), or to a trust established for that child's benefit;

- transfers of an individual's home to the spouse, a child under age 21, a blind or disabled child of any age, a sibling who has an equity interest in the home and who resided in it for at least one year prior to the institutionalization of the applicant, or a child who resided in the home for at least two (2) years and who provided services to the applicant that delayed institutionalization;

- transfers where the assets have been returned;

- transfers where the state determines that a penalty would result in undue hardship; or

- transfers to a trust, under certain circumstances, in some states.

G.   Are Transfers to or by a Trust Subject to the Trust Transfer Penalty Rules?

It depends. As itemized and set forth below, the transfer penalty rules impose a penalty upon certain, but not all, transfers of assets into and from certain kinds of trusts. **The transfer penalty rules apply to and impose a penalty on transfers to and from an irrevocable trust, pooled trust and income-only trust.** The rules do not apply to revocable trusts, trusts for the disabled under age 65, nor Miller trusts, each of which is considered an **exempt trust**.

- **Revocable Trust**. The principal of this trust is not subject to the transfer of assets rules. This is also true for the establishment of a revocable trust. Moreover, payments from the trust are subject to transfer rules and penalties only to the extent payments are made to or for the benefit of someone other than the individual applying for or receiving Medicaid.

- **Irrevocable Trust**. Transfers of assets into an irrevocable trust are penalized if the assets cannot be paid under any circumstances to the individual Medicaid applicant. Any portion of the assets which could be paid to or used for the benefit of the individual creating the trust is outside the purview of the penalty rules. Payments from this trust are penalized if they are not actually paid to or for the benefit of the individual whose assets established the trust but are paid to or for the benefit of other individuals.

- **Trusts for the Disabled**. Transfer rules expressly exempt transfers to trusts established for a disabled child and to a trust established for disabled individuals under age 65. In addition, it would appear that, as in the case of transfers that are made outright, no penalty would be incurred if assets transferred to the trust are returned to the individual.

- **Miller Trust**. The transfer of income into this trust will not be penalized if and to the extent that the trust instrument provides that such income will be used to pay for medical care provided to the individual. The transfer of any income not used (e.g., income which exceeds the amount paid for these medical services) will be penalized.

- **Pooled Trust**. This trust is not exempt from the transfer of assets rules. However, a transfer to a pooled trust is exempt if the transfer is made by a disabled person under age 65 at the time the trust is established.

- **Income-only Trust**. The value of the trust principal will be treated, for transfer penalty purposes, as a transfer of assets for less than fair market value, and therefore is subject to transfer penalty.

Chapter 4   **Transfer of Assets Penalty Rules**
                                                                                              (continued)

H.   **Is the Transfer Penalty Applicable to All Medicaid Services?**

No. **The transfer penalty rule does not apply to all Medicaid services, <u>only</u> to the following designated services**: (i) <u>nursing home services</u>, (ii) <u>waivered services</u> (under a Federal waiver requested by a state of the Federal government), <u>and</u> (iii) at the option of a state, <u>home health care</u>. Thus, <u>in New York state, for example, the transfer penalty rules do not apply to home health services</u>. (In New York, a Medicaid applicant who is not institutionalized and who is eligible for home health care is entitled to obtain non-waivered services, notwithstanding he/she may have made transfers of his/her assets, without any concern for the transfer penalty rules. The penalty transfer rules do not apply to the non-waivered services.)

The designated services affected by the transfer penalty rules differ in the case of institutionalized and non-institutionalized persons:

1. **For institutionalized individuals** – designated services include the following:

    - Nursing home services;

    - A level of care in any institution equivalent to that of nursing facility services such as skilled nursing or custodial care in a hospital while awaiting transfer to a nursing home; and

    - Home or community-based care authorized under the waiver program (waivered services).

2. **For non-institutionalized persons – <u>only</u> in the case <u>where the state has elected to apply the transfer penalty rules to non-institutionalized persons</u>** will the following designated services be covered and affected by the transfer penalty rule:

    - Home health care;

    - Any other type of remedial care recognized under state law specified by the Secretary of HHS;

    - Community-supported living arrangements related to services to assist a developmentally disabled individual in activities of daily living to permit them to live in their own home, apartment, family home or rental unit furnished in a <u>community-supported living</u> setting. Services include personal assistance, training, and a twenty-four- (24)hour emergency response system.

III. DOES MEDICAID OFFER HOME CARE SERVICES TO MEDICAID ELIGIBLES?

Yes. Medicaid offers eligible persons a wide variety of benefits and services, some of which are expressly selected by a particular state, according to Federal and state agreements.

A. What Medicaid Services Are Federally Required?

- inpatient and outpatient hospital services (except in institutions for the mentally ill or the developmentally disabled);
- laboratory and x-ray services;
- physician's services;
- medical or surgical dental services;
- transportation to medical appointments; and
- **home health services**, provided by a certified home health agency, consisting of part-time and intermittent nursing, medical supplies, and home health aide services for those states that have opted to cover nursing home services.

B. What Medicaid Home Care Benefits Are Optional to States?

Optional benefits selected by each state Medicaid program run the gamut. They may include the following home care benefits:

- Non-medical personal care services;
- in-home physical, occupational, speech, and audiology services; and
- private duty nursing.

In addition, states may obtain permission from the Federal government to offer experimental services through so-called Medicaid waivers.

C. Which Home and Community-based Long-term Care Services Can a State Offer on a Waivered Basis?

Home and community-based long-term care waiver services are intended to enable a homebound person to remain at home and delay or obviate the need for nursing home care. In some states this service is called

| Chapter 4 | Medicaid Home Services (continued) |

"nursing home without walls." Variations of the services listed below may be available:

- Case management services;
- Homemaker or housekeeping services;
- Nursing care;
- Home health aide services;
- Personal care services;
- Adult day care;
- Respite care; and
- Any other services at the state's option (such as chore assistance, transportation, meal preparation, home modification, home maintenance, and social work services).

D. What Is "Personal" Care under Medicaid?

Personal care means some or total assistance with personal hygiene, dressing and feeding; nutritional and environmental support functions, and health related tasks. The services may include:

- Basic personal care and grooming, including bathing, hair care and assistance with clothing;
- Assistance with bladder and bowel requirements, including helping the patient to the bathroom or with a bed pan;
- Helping with medications that are ordinarily self-administered;
- Assisting with food, nutrition, and diet, including preparing meals, if incidental to a medical need; and
- Performing household services if related to a medical need and if they are essential to the patient's health and comfort at home.

E. Are Personal Care Aides Trained and Supervised?

It depends.

States that provide optional Medicaid personal care through personal care aides or home attendants usually require them to be trained in personal care skills. But personal care aides have less medical-oriented training and skills than home health aides (as described in Chapter 1, section II.C). However, as a practical matter, the distinction is blurred between the personal care services which are performed by personal care aides and the slightly more skilled services provided by home health aides. As a rule, the tasks of the home attendant or personal care aide are not as intensely supervised as the tasks performed by home health aides.

NOTE: The home care agency that provides <u>non-medical personal care aides</u> does not have to be a certified home health agency (in contrast to providers of medically oriented home health services under Medicare and Medicaid, which must be certified home health agencies).

F. Are There Medicaid Qualifying Conditions for Home Health Care?

Yes. Unlike Medicare, Medicaid does not require that patients be homebound, or that they need part-time intermittent skilled nursing services or therapy, as a condition to obtaining home care. State law may impose limits on the number of hours of home health care, and the state may deny the delivery of home care under state law, if other, more cost-effective services would address the patient's needs (including nursing facility care, or other community-based services). <u>The following conditions must be satisfied in order to obtain Medicaid-covered home heath care</u>:

- The patient must be eligible for Medicaid coverage under the state plan;

- Home heath services must be provided in the recipient's home;

- The services must be prescribed by the person's physician;

- The mandated medical home care services must be provided by a certified home health agency and must be performed by a properly trained person (not family member); and

- The care must be supervised by a registered nurse who must visit the patient every three months.

G. Does Medicaid Impose Qualifying Conditions for Personal Care Services?

Yes.

Chapter 4   **Medicaid Home Services**
                                                                                                                      (continued)

<u>Medicaid personal care services</u> generally include the following requirements:

- The **application for personal care services** must be based on the order of a physician or other professional designated by the state. The physician's order form must include the patient's medical condition and the patient's need for assistance with personal care services. The completed and signed order form must be submitted to the Medicaid agency.

- If the patient is not receiving Medicaid, a separate **Medicaid application** should be submitted to the state agency, together with the home care application and the physician's order.

- The state Medicaid agency usually requires a **nursing assessment**, which will recommend what services are needed by the patient, for a designated number of days per week and hours per day.

- The state Medicaid agency generally also conducts a **social assessment** of the need for personal care services, which includes an assessment of the home environment and its suitability for the delivery of home care.

- The state Medicaid agency may also conduct an **assessment of other services and efficiencies** to ensure that the most cost-effective package of services is being used in every plan of care.

- A **fiscal assessment** may be conducted by the state agency to determine whether the cost of home care exceeds the cost of skilled nursing facility care in the patient's community.

H.   **How Does One Find Out about Individual State Programs?**

In order to find out what Medicaid services and benefits are available in a particular state, individuals are advised to contact their **local office on aging** for more detailed information about the eligibility rules and benefits in their community. Other sources for information and advice are **elder law attorneys, lawyers** who specialize in estate planning with a view toward lifetime planning for long-term care, and **geriatric care managers** who are **social workers, nurses, or psychologists** specializing in care management, daily money management and long-distance care giving. Application for Medicaid home care and information about Medicaid home care may also be obtained from **local home care agencies.**

IV. CAN MEDICAID RECOVER COSTS OF MEDICAL ASSISTANCE?

Yes in certain instances.

1. Liens on Real Property of Medicaid Recipient

State Medicaid programs are authorized, but not required, to place liens on property of Medicaid recipients in two limited circumstances:

- For benefits incorrectly paid, pursuant to a judgment from a court; and

- On real property for a permanently institutionalized individuals when the state has determined, after an opportunity for a hearing, that the individual cannot be reasonably expected to return home.

The term permanently institutionalized is not defined in the statute. No liens can be placed on a life estate of a Medicaid recipient. Medicaid does not consider a life estate as a countable resource.

Liens cannot be imposed on **homesteads** if any of the following persons are lawfully residing in the institutionalized individual's home:

- His/her spouse; his/her child who is under age 21, blind or disabled or;

- A sibling as long as he/she has an equity interest in the home and has resided there for at least one year prior to the institutionalized individual's entry into a nursing facility.

The lien on real property will dissolve when the Medicaid recipient is discharged from the institution and returns home.

2. Medicaid Recovery from Community Spouse (Spousal Refusal).

When a community spouse has excess resources over and above the community spouse's resource allowance and the community spouse refuses (Spousal Refusal) to turn over his/her resources available to meet the Medicaid recipient's needs, States may and are likely to seek recovery of costs expended on the Medicaid recipient's care.

3. Medicaid Recovery from Estate of a Deceased Recipient.

Federal law mandates that each state place into effect an estate recovery program, which provides for recovery from a Medicaid recipient of medical assistance for him/her.

Estate recovery can occur: (i) only after the death of the Medicaid recipient age 55 or older who received Medicaid care in a medical institution (e.g., nursing home or at home for waivered home and community-based services); and (ii) only if there is no surviving spouse, disabled children or children under age 21. The estate of a Medicaid recipient is sheltered from recovery in whole or in part if the recipient purchased a long-term care insurance policy under the Robert Wood Johnson program (see Chapter 9, section XVII).

The term "estate" refers to all real and personal property and other assets included within an individual's estate under state probate law. In connection with its recovery program, Medicaid permits states to use a broader definition of the term to include whether or not the asset is the subject of probate, any real or personal property and other assets in which an individual had an interest at the time of death such as an interest in jointly owned property. The term "estate" does not include special powers of appointment under trusts which are expressly stated not to be an asset conveyed to a survivor.

The amount of an annuity will be subject to estate recovery upon the death of the Medicaid recipient unless (i) there is a surviving spouse or disabled or minor child or (ii) the annuity is sheltered because of his/her participation in the Robert Wood Johnson Program (see section VII below).

V. WHAT ARE THE DUE PROCESS RIGHTS FOR APPEALING MEDICAID DECISIONS?

Since Medicaid is a public agency, it is possible to appeal an erroneous Medicaid decision, according to well-established due process rights available to applicants and Medicaid beneficiaries.

Due process refers to procedures that must be followed to enable a person to appeal an erroneous Medicaid decision. The types of decisions that can be appealed are broad and include: a mistaken denial of Medicaid eligibility; a denial, suspension, or termination of home care benefits; the amount of home care that has been approved; or, any other decision made by the Medicaid agency that the patient believes is incorrect.

Due process rights start with the submission of an application in writing to the state-approved agency. If an application is denied for whatever reason, the applicant must be given the opportunity to have the Medicaid decision reviewed by an independent person to determine whether it was accurate or not. Due process rights include the following:

- **The right to a written notice** with respect to the person's claim and the reason for the decision; generally, the state or the local agency must mail the notice at least ten (10) days before benefits are reduced or discontinued.;

- **The right to request a fair hearing** within a reasonable time, following the receipt of the notice (usually ninety (90) days from the date of he mailing of the notice);

- **The right to a hearing** conducted by a hearing officer (usually a lawyer) who was not involved in the initial decision and who must be impartial;

- **The right to a written hearing decision**;

- If the decision continues to be adverse, **the right to appeal in a state court**; and

- **The right to continue to receive benefits pending the outcome of the hearing.** This right is only available if services had already started and the request for the hearing was made within a prescribed number of days of the mailing date of the notice.

VI. CAN MEDICAID MANDATE MANAGED CARE?

Yes.

The Balanced Budget Act of 1997 amended the Social Security Act with the addition of Section 1932, titled Provisions Relating to Managed Care. **This authorizes states to require individuals eligible for Medicaid medical assistance**, subject to some exceptions noted below, **to enroll in a managed care entity**.

A **"managed care entity"** refers to either a **Medicaid managed care organization**, or **primary care case management**. These two terms are defined in H below.

In a managed care entity, a primary care physician coordinates and approves an array of services in addition to providing primary care services. Usually, physicians are paid case management fees in addition to their regular fee-for-service payments for the primary care services they provide.

A. Is Anyone Eligible for Medicaid Exempt from Mandatory Enrollment in Managed Care?

Children under age 19 with special needs (e.g., children receiving foster care) and dual eligible individuals are exempt from mandatory enrollment but may voluntarily enroll.

B. Does an Individual Have a Choice of Managed Care Entities?

A state must give individuals a choice of at least two (2) managed care entities or primary care case managers. In rural areas, eligible individuals must be permitted to: receive such assistance through no fewer than two (2) physicians or case managers to the extent that they are available to provide such assistance in the area; and obtain Medicaid medical assistance from any other provider under appropriate circumstances as set forth by CMS regulations.

C. Are Medicaid Recipients Guaranteed Eligibility to a Managed Care Entity?

Individuals enrolled with a Medicaid managed care organization or a primary care case manager are guaranteed Medicaid eligibility for six (6) months from the date of enrollment, even if his/her eligibility otherwise terminates during that period.

Chapter 4 — Medicaid-mandated Managed Care (continued)

D. What Are an Individual's Rights When Terminating or Changing Enrollment in a Medicaid Managed Care Organization?

An individual must be permitted to terminate or change enrollment at any time for cause and may do so without cause during the ninety- (90) day period beginning on the day he/she receives notice of enrollment and at least once annually thereafter. States must establish notice of termination requirements as well as a method for determining enrollment priorities in the event a managed care organization does not have the capacity to enroll all individuals seeking enrollment.

The state must establish a default enrollment process for enrolling any person who does not choose a managed care organization during a state's specified enrollment period. This process must provide for enrollment in a managed care organization that maintains existing provider-individual relationships or has contracted with providers that have traditionally served Medicaid recipients.

E. What Information Must Be Provided to a Medicaid Managed Care Participant?

Each state or managed care organization must provide all enrollment notices and other information in easily understood form. Upon request, each Medicaid managed care organization must make available to enrollees and potential enrollees information concerning providers, enrollees' responsibilities and rights, grievance and **appeals procedures** and information on covered items and services.

A state requiring enrollment in a managed care organization must annually provide Medicaid recipients a list identifying available managed care organizations, their benefits, cost-sharing, service area, quality and performance.

F. What Access to Emergency Services Do Medicaid Managed Care Participants Have?

Each Medicaid managed care organization or primary care case manager must provide coverage for emergency services without regard to prior authorization or the emergency care provider's contractual relationship with the organization or manager. Emergency services are inpatient and outpatient medical services that are rendered by a provider qualified to

| Chapter 4 | Medicaid-mandated Managed Care (continued) |

furnish them and that are needed to evaluate or stabilize an emergency medical condition.

An emergency medical condition manifests itself by acute symptoms of sufficient severity, including severe pain, such that a lay person can reasonably expect the absence of immediate medical attention to seriously jeopardize the health of an individual, or in the case of a pregnant woman, the health of the woman or her unborn child; or result in serious impairment to bodily functions or serious dysfunction of any bodily organ or part.

G. Can a Medicare Managed Care Organization Restrict Enrollee-Provider Communications?

A Medicaid managed care organization may not prohibit or otherwise restrict a health professional from advising the enrollee who is a patient of that professional about the enrollee's health status or the medical care and treatment of his/her conditions, regardless of whether benefits for such care or treatment are provided under the organization's contract.

H. How Are Medicaid Managed Care Organization and Primary Care Case Management Defined?

1. **Medicaid managed care organization**

The entities considered a Medicaid managed care organization are:

- a health maintenance organization;
- an eligible organization with a contract under Section 1876 of the Social Security Act;
- a Medicare Advantage organization with a contract under Part C of Title XVIII of Medicare;
- a provider-sponsored organization; or
- any other public or private organization that meets the requirements of Section 1902(w) of the Social Security Act.

2. **Primary care case management**

One type of arrangement under which Medicaid provides managed care is called primary care case management (PCCM). Under PCCM arrangements, a primary care physician coordinates and

Chapter 4

Medicaid-mandated Managed Care
(continued)

approves an array of services in addition to providing primary care services. In most PCCM systems, physicians are paid case management fees in addition to their regular fee-for-service payment for the primary care services they provide. In a few PCCM systems, physicians are placed at financial risk for some services, usually ambulatory care. They may determine the level of their Medicaid caseloads, up to a state-specified limit.

VII. CAN STATE LONG-TERM PARTNERSHIP PROGRAMS AFFECT MEDICAID INCOME AND/OR RESOURCE ELIGIBILITY STANDARDS?

Yes, in the case of resources.

No, in the case of income.

Several states following pilot projects funded by grants from the Robert Wood Johnson Foundation have enacted long-term care insurance (LTCI) programs integrating the purchase by an individual of LTCI with his/her eligibility for Medicaid. <u>California, Connecticut, Indiana, Iowa and New York</u> approved such plans in 1993. Federal law (COBRA 1993) previously banned extension of this type of program to other states. The Deficit Reduction Act of 2005 (DRA) authorized all other states to adopt the program.

According to this plan linking LTCI with Medicaid eligibility rules, <u>if and when private insurance benefits are exhausted, the **resources** of policyholders are **not counted** in whole or in part in determining their Medicaid eligibility. However, all of their **income** will be counted. Under the New York plan, a person who purchases a LTCI policy may establish his/her eligibility for Medicaid when the insurance benefits run out</u> and thereby **shelter some or all assets from recovery** by Medicaid. <u>In the four (4) other states, a purchase of an LTCI policy will shelter assets on a dollar-for-dollar basis</u>. The individual purchaser is able to retain an amount of assets **free from Medicaid recovery** equal to the amount of LTCI purchased.

The DRA provides that <u>states now may amend their Medicaid plans</u> to include qualified long-term care partnership programs that disregard assets or resources equal to the amount of insurance benefit payments made to or on behalf of a beneficiary under a long-term care insurance policy if the statutorily specified requirements are met regarding the insured and the policy. Under DRA, the programs in California, Connecticut, Indiana Iowa, and New York are "grandfathered" into the new provisions so long as the Secretary of HHS determines that each state's consumer protection standards are no less stringent than the standards applicable as of December 31, 2005. Other states that wish to offer the program may amend their Medicaid statutes to provide for the program.

Chapter 4

State Long-Term Care Partnership Programs
(continued)

A. **What Are the Requirements of a Qualified State Long-term Care Insurance Policy?**

In order to qualify as a "**qualified state long-term care insurance partnership policy**," the policy must satisfy seven (7) requirements:

- The insured must be a resident of the state at the time coverage first becomes effective;

- The policy must be a qualified long-term care insurance policy as defined in IRC Section 7702B(b);

- The policy must meet nine (9) specified sections of the Long-Term Care Insurance Model Act and nineteen (19) specified sections of the Model Regulations of the National Association of Insurance Commissioners (NAIC);

- The policy must provide for "compound annual inflation protection" for persons under age 61 as of the purchase date and must also provide "some level of inflation protection" for persons between the ages of 61 and 75. From age 76 on, inflation protection is optional;

- The state Medicaid agency must provide information and technical assistance to the state insurance department to make sure that agents selling long-term care insurance receive training and demonstrate understanding of the partnership long-term care insurance policies and how they relate to other private and public coverage of long-term care;

- The insurer must provide regular reports to the Secretary of HHS regarding the performance of the program; and

- The state may not impose requirements on partnership policies that are not imposed on all long-term care policies.

CHAPTER 5

ORIGINAL MEDICARE
PRESCRIPTION DRUGS (PART D)

I. WHAT IS THE MEDICARE PRESCRIPTION DRUG PROGRAM?

Prescription drug coverage benefits are available to everyone eligible for Medicare **Part D** coverage (see section III.A below) under a newly enacted **Medicare Part D Program** of Title XVIII of the Social Security Act (the "Act") (Section 101 of the Medicare Modernization Act (MMA), effective December 8, 2003). The Centers for Medicare and Medicaid Services (CMS) has overall responsibility for implementing the Medicare Part D prescription drug benefit program.

The Act provides for premium and subsidies of prescription drug coverage for certain individuals with low incomes and limited resources. The purpose of the subsidy program is to assist Medicare beneficiaries with limited financial means, to pay for Medicare prescription drug coverage under Medicare Part D. Individuals with low incomes and limited resources may be eligible for this subsidy (sometimes referred to as **extra help subsidy**) to help pay for monthly premiums, coinsurances and the annual deductible under Medicare Part D.

Enrollment in Part D requires the beneficiary to take affirmative steps to enroll and get Part D coverage. He/she must first choose a drug plan from the options available in his/her area, and then must enroll through the plan he/she chooses. He/she must file a separate application for the extra help subsidy either with the state Medicaid agency or with Social Security.

Medicare beneficiaries are able to obtain qualified prescription drug coverage either through **(i) <u>Stand-alone prescription drug plans</u>**, or <u>**alternative prescription drug coverage**</u>, available to enrollees in Original Medicare, or (ii) <u>**a comprehensive Medicare Advantage plan**</u> available to Medicare-eligibles who enroll in Medicare Advantage plans (see Chapter 7). The prescription drug coverage is operated through private insurance entities that contract with CMS. **This chapter relates only to stand-alone prescription drug plans (PDP) or alternative prescription drug coverage available to Original Medicare-eligibles.**

An individual is eligible for the Medicare prescription drug program if he or she is entitled to Medicare Part A and/or enrolled in Medicare Part B. The benefits are voluntary.

Chapter 5   **Introduction**
                                                                                                                       (continued)

Insurance companies are no longer able to sell existing Medigap policies that provide drug coverage to Medicare beneficiaries who are enrolled in or eligible for Medicare outpatient prescription drug coverage. They are, however, able to renew the Medigap drug policies issued prior to January 1, 2006 for beneficiaries who do not opt for the Medicare PDP; their Medigap policy will be modified to eliminate drug coverage, and premiums will be adjusted. Beneficiaries with the new Medicare drug coverage can purchase Medigap policies that do not cover drugs.

Medicare may not negotiate drug discounts. The MMA prohibits the government from negotiating discounts on drug purchases or otherwise interfering in drug pricing decisions.

Medicaid does not cover Part D drugs.

II. WHAT IS A PART D DRUG UNDER THE MEDICARE PART D PROGRAM?

A Part D drug is a drug that is approved by the U.S. Food and Drug Administration, for which a prescription is required, and for which payment is required under Medicare. Biological products, including insulin and insulin supplies (syringes, needles, alcohol swabs and gauge) and smoking cessation drugs are also covered under Part D. The Medicare Modernization Act (MMA) excludes from coverage those categories of drugs for which Medicare payment is optional, such as drugs for weight gain, barbiturates, benzodiazepines and over-the-counter medications. MMA also excludes from Part D coverage those drugs for which payment could be made under Medicare Part A or Part B.

A plan's drug **formulary** must include at least one (but often two) drugs in each approved category and class. All drug plan sponsors must establish an **exceptions** process whereby individuals enrolled in a drug plan can seek a non-formulary drug, or to have a covered drug assigned to a lower tier to reduce their cost-sharing.

CMS has developed **appeals** procedures which ensure that enrollees quickly receive decisions regarding medically necessary medications. Pharmacies will distribute or post notices that instruct enrollees to contact their Medicare prescription drug plan if they need a certain drug and the pharmacist informs them that the drug is not included in the plan's formulary. **The plans may change their formularies any time** upon giving a sixty- (60) day notice to the enrollee, his/her proscribing physician, pharmacist and CMS, of formulary changes. The notice must explain how an enrollee may request an **exception**. The prescribing doctor must show that all of the drugs on any tier of the plan's formulary for treatment of the same condition would not be as effective or would have adverse consequences. Denial of an exception request constitutes an unfavorable coverage determination. The plan must act within the time frames for standard coverage determinations (72 hours) or expedited coverage determinations (24 hours), depending on which standards are met. **A beneficiary may appeal the denial of an exception request through the statutory appeals process.**

III. WHO IS ELIGIBLE TO ENROLL IN THE PART D PRESCRIPTION DRUG PROGRAM, AND WHEN CAN AN INDIVIDUAL ELIGIBLE FOR PART D ENROLL?

A. Who Is Eligible?

A **Part D-eligible** individual is someone entitled to benefits under Part A <u>or</u> enrolled in Part B. Persons with end-stage renal disease (ESRD) are excluded from taking part in the program (but an individual who develops ESRD already enrolled in a prescription drug plan may continue that plan). Persons who wish to enroll in an outpatient prescription drug plan (PDP) cannot enroll in a Medicare Advantage (MA) plan except that an enrollee in a Medical Savings Account may obtain prescription drug coverage through enrollment in a PDP. <u>Individuals in Original Medicare can only join a Medicare PDP</u>. If they disenroll from Original Medicare, then the individual may join an MA plan that includes drug coverage.

Note: <u>If a Part D-eligible individual has prescription drug coverage from a former or current employer or union, he/she should contact his/her benefits administrator before making any changes to his/her coverage. If he/she joins a Medicare PDP or Medicare Advantage plan, such individual and/or his/her family may lose their employer or union coverage</u>.

B. In Order to Obtain Part D Drugs, Is It Necessary to Enroll in a Prescription Drug Plan?

Yes.

Participation requires enrollment in a PDP. In order for Medicare beneficiaries to take part in the Medicare Part D prescription drug program, it is incumbent upon them to take affirmative steps to enroll in a PDP. These plans are offered by insurance companies and other private companies and cover both generic and brand-name drugs. The plans serving the fee-for-service Medicare population ("Original Medicare") are called **prescription drug plans (PDP), also known as stand-alone plans**, and those serving Medicare Advantage enrollees are called **Medicare Advantage prescription drug plans (MA-PDP)**. The beneficiary must first choose a drug plan from the options available in his/her area. Then, the beneficiary must enroll through the plan that he/she chooses. If the beneficiary is eligible as a **subsidy-eligible individual**, for a low-income subsidy, he/she must file a second affirmation.

Individuals who are eligible for Medicare and Medicaid (dual eligibles), and who do not choose their own PDP during their initial enrollment period, are not automatically assigned into a drug plan. However, they are **automatically eligible** for a **continuous special enrollment period**.

C. **When Are the Periods to Enroll for Medicare Part D Coverage?**

There are **three (3) coverage enrollment periods**: (i) the initial enrollment period; (ii) the annual coordinated election period; and (iii) special enrollment periods.

1. <u>**Initial Enrollment Period**</u>. The initial enrollment period for individuals who are first eligible to enroll in Part D, corresponds to the initial enrollment period for Part B, i.e., the seven- (7) month period running from three (3) months before the month the individual first becomes eligible and ending three (3) months after the first month of eligibility.

    The initial open enrollment in Part D runs from November 15 through December 31, when Original Medicare beneficiaries may switch from Original Medicare to a Medicare Advantage plan or enroll in a stand-alone plan if they have not previously done so. **Rephrased**: Beneficiaries may remain in Original Medicare and receive prescription drug coverage through **stand-alone prescription drug plans (drug-only plan)**, or join a **Medicare Advantage plan** that offers comprehensive benefits, including outpatient prescription drugs. Beneficiaries who become eligible for Medicare may enroll in a Part D plan <u>when</u> they become eligible for Part A or Part B benefits (three (3) months before an individual reaches age 65, until three (3) months after the month he/she turns 65). If an individual does join when first eligible, he/she can join between November 15 and December 31 of each year; and coverage will be effective January of the following year.

2. <u>**Annual Coordinated Enrollment Period**</u>. The annual coordinated enrollment period corresponds to the annual coordinated enrollment period for Medicare Part C and runs from November 15 through December 31.

3. <u>**Special Enrollment Periods**</u>. Individuals may be eligible for a special enrollment period, if:

Chapter 5   **Eligibility and Enrollment**
                                                                                (continued)

- They did not enroll in Part D during their initial enrollment because they had other prescription drug coverage deemed to be **creditable coverage**, and they lose the creditable coverage;

- They were given incorrect information concerning the creditable coverage status of their other prescription drug coverage;

- They were given incorrect enrollment information by a Federal employee;

- They have Medicare and full Medicaid coverage (full-benefit dual eligibility) or are enrolled in Medical Savings Account program;

- They move out of a plan's service area;

- Their PDP's contract with Medicare is terminated;

- They enrolled in a MA-PDP during the first year of eligibility and want to return to traditional Medicare and a PDP; or,

- They move into or out of a nursing home.

D.   **What Is the Effective Date of Enrollment Coverage?**

Enrollment coverage becomes effective:

- The same month that Part A and/or Part B coverage becomes effective for individuals who enroll before their month of entitlement to Part A or enrollment in Part B;

- The first day of the next calendar month after enrollment for individuals who enroll after the first month of entitlement for Part A or enrollment in Part B;

- The following January 1, for individuals who enroll during the annual coordinated enrollment period; and

- At the time specified by CMS for individuals who enroll during a special enrollment period.

Enrollment of full-benefit dual eligible individuals is effective the first day of the month for: 1) the individual who is Medicaid-eligible and subsequently becomes newly eligible for Part D; or (2) the individual who is eligible for Part D, and subsequently becomes newly eligible for Medicaid.

E. Can an Enrollee of a Prescription Drug Plan Change Plans Mid-Year?

Yes, but only in the following instances:

1. <u>During the annual coordinated enrollment period</u>. All beneficiaries may switch plans once during the annual coordinated enrollment period, which runs from November 15 to December 31. Enrollment becomes effective on January 1 of the next year.

2. <u>During special enrollment periods</u>. Beneficiaries may be eligible to change plans mid-year if they qualify for a special enrollment period described in section C.3 above.

Individuals who enroll in a PDP are locked in to their plan for the remainder of the calendar year, even though the plan in which they enroll may change the formulary or **cost-sharing** arrangements during the year. Enrollees in PDPs must wait until the next annual enrollment period to switch plans, with enrollment in the new plan becoming effective on January 1 of the following year. Full-benefit dual eligibles are automatically eligible for a continuous special enrollment period and therefore are not ever locked into a prescription drug plan.

F. Is There a Penalty for Late Enrollment?

Yes. A beneficiary who does not enroll in a Part D plan within sixty-three (63) days of his/her initial enrollment period, and who does not have other **creditable** prescription drug coverage, must pay a late penalty if he/she subsequently enrolls in a Part D plan. The penalty is assessed at one (1) percent of the national average premium for each month of delayed enrollment for the remainder of the time in which the beneficiary is enrolled in a Part D plan. Thus, a beneficiary who first becomes eligible for Part D at age 65, but who delays enrolling until age 70 may be assessed a sixty (60) percent penalty on his/her premium (5 years x 12 months x 1%). Since the penalty is based on a percentage of the average premium each year, the dollar value of the penalty changes as the national average premium changes.

Late enrollment penalties will not be imposed if a beneficiary maintains **creditable coverage** (i.e., other coverage comparable to Part D coverage such as MA-PDP or stand-alone PDP coverage; Veterans Administration coverage; and most employer- (or union) sponsored retiree plans). Should a beneficiary's existing drug coverage end or change and thereby cease to be "creditable," he/she has up to sixty-three (63) days to enroll in a Medicare PDP.

Chapter 5 — Costs of Prescription Drug Plans

IV. WHAT ARE THE COSTS OF THE PRESCRIPTION DRUG PLANS?

MMA established a **standard drug plan** and **alternative prescription drug coverage** for Part D-eligibles. The **cost-sharing** benefits of the Part D drugs under these two plans are set forth below.

A. What Are the Costs of the Standard Drug Plan?

The MMA established a standard drug plan that Part D plans may offer. It consists of the following salient features:

1. A monthly **premium** (which amounts to approximately $25.00 and varies depending on the plan chosen).

2. A yearly **deductible** of $275 (2008).

3. Twenty-five (25) percent of the yearly drug costs of $2,235 (2008), representing the costs between $275 and $2,510 (**initial coverage limit**) which amounts to $558.75. The plan pays the other seventy-five (75) percent (plan cost-share) which represents $1,676.25 (2008).

4. One-hundred (100) percent of the next **additional out-of-pocket expenses** of $3,216.25 (2008) in drug costs (sometimes referred to as the "**doughnut hole**" or "**coverage gap**"). The beneficiary must pay the plan's premiums while in the coverage gap.

5. After having spent $4,050 (2008) out-of-pocket expenses (**out-of-pocket threshold**) – the total of the items 2 ($275), 3 ($558.75) and 4 ($3,216.25) above) – the beneficiary thereafter will have **catastrophic coverage**. This means the individual during this entire period of coverage will only have to pay $2.25 co-payment for a generic or preferred Part D drug and $5.60 for other drugs or five (5) percent coinsurance, whichever is greater. The plan pays for the rest.

The deductible, initial coverage limit, out-of-pocket expenses, and annual out-of-pocket expenses threshold are indexed for inflation each year.

A breakdown of the foregoing payments by a beneficiary totaling $4,050 (2008) is outlined in the table below.

Chapter 5   **Costs of Prescription Drug Plans**
(continued)

Annual Deductible	$275.00
25% Co-pay of costs between the $275 deductible and the **initial coverage limit** of $2,510	$558.75
Subtotal (annual deductible + co-pay)	$833.75
Additional out-of-pocket expenses (donut hole)	$3,216.25
Out-of-pocket threshold	$4,050.00

B.   What Are the Costs of an Alternative Prescription Drug Coverage Plan?

Part D drug plans are not required to offer the standard benefit, but can offer **alternative prescription drug coverage**. <u>Alternative coverage must be actuarially equivalent to the standard coverage</u>. In an actuarially equivalent plan, the cost-sharing varies through the use of such mechanisms as tiered co-payments. However, a plan that offers an alternative benefit package cannot impose a higher annual deducible ($275 in 2008) or require a higher out-of-pocket threshold ($4,050 in 2008) than required by the standard benefit. Plans can offer <u>enhanced alternative coverage</u> that may include changes to the deductible and the initial coverage limit, though the deductible cannot be higher than $275 (2008). **Enhanced alternative coverage** under Part D might include coverage of some drugs that are excluded under Part D, or that are in the coverage gap (doughnut hole). A PDP that wants to offer a drug plan with enhanced alternative coverage in a service area must also offer a PDP with the basic benefit prescription package in that area.

<u>Note</u>: Part D-eligibles are offered a wide variety of drug plans which must abide by the requirements of the foregoing coverages, but may present variations such as **gap coverage insurance**, no deductibles, higher or lower premiums and/or co-payments, etc. For example:

- A plan may require a relatively higher premium, say, of $64.10 per month, with no deductibles and doughnut hole gap coverage. However, the insurance typically covers only generic drugs.

Chapter 5   **Costs of Prescription Drug Plans**
                                                                                                 (continued)

- A plan may provide for a far lower premium of $16.40 per month, but would end up costing $250 more by the end of the year – and a full $1,100 compared with the plan mentioned above.

- A plan that limits the quantity of drugs a patient may get each month.

- A plan may require prior authorization for certain drugs.

- A plan may add extra levels of co-pays or move drugs from one amount of co-pay to another.

The cheapest plan is not necessarily the best. Among things to consider are whether a plan carries a deductible, what it charges for co-payments on individual drugs, whether it covers drugs in the doughnut hole, the amount of the premiums, and whether there are restrictions on some drugs.

C.   **Are Subsidies Available to Help Low-income Individuals Pay for Part D Drug Coverage?** (see also section VI below)

The MMA provides for deductible, premium and cost-sharing subsidies of prescription drug coverage for certain individuals with low incomes and limited resources (called **extra help**). The purpose of the subsidy program is to assist Medicare beneficiaries with limited financial means to pay for Medicare prescription drug coverage under Medicare Part D.

To qualify for extra help with prescription drug costs, individuals must meet specific income and resource limits (for more details see section VI (A.1)). Resources include savings and stocks, but not an individual's home or car. If an individual qualifies, he/she will receive help paying for the Medicare drug plan's monthly premium, yearly deductible, and prescription co-payments. Subsidy-eligible individuals do not have a coverage gap.

An individual <u>automatically qualifies</u> for extra help if he/she has Medicare and:

Chapter 5   Costs of Prescription Drug Plans
(continued)

- Has, or becomes eligible for, Medicaid benefits; (see section VI.A(2));

- Gets help from his/her state Medicaid program paying Medicare premiums (i.e., the individual belongs to a Medicare savings program) (see section VI.A(3)); or

- Receives Supplemental Security Income (SSI) benefits without Medicaid (see section VI.A(3)).

If an individual lives in Alaska or Hawaii, or pays more than half of the living expenses of dependent family members, income limits are higher. Puerto Rico, the Virgin Islands, Guam, the Northern Mariana Islands, and American Samoa have their own rules for providing extra help to their residents.

Chapter 5 Joining a PDP

V. HOW DOES A PERSON ELIGIBLE FOR PART D JOIN A PDP?

In its handbook (*Medicare and You 2008*), CMS suggests the following steps:

1. Get personalized help comparing Medicare prescription drug coverage.

2. Visit www.medicare.gov on the web. Select "Compare Medicare Prescription Drug Plans."

3. Call 1-800-MEDICARE (1-800-633-4227). TTY users should call 1-877-486-2048.

4. Call a State Health Insurance Assistance Program.

5. An individual should have available his/her Medicare card, a list of drugs and their dosage, and the name of the pharmacy he/she uses.

6. Consider the following factors:

    - <u>Drug coverage</u>. Check to see if the plan covers prescription drugs needed by the individual. If a drug is on the plan's list, there may be special rules for filling the prescription. The list can change during the year because drug therapies change, and new drugs and medical knowledge become available.

    - <u>Cost</u>. See how much an individual's prescription drugs would cost in each drug plan.

    - <u>Convenience</u>. Medicare drug plans must contract with pharmacies in an individual's area. Check with the plan to make sure the pharmacies in the plan are the ones the individual wants to use.

7. Steps to take to join a PDP:

    - <u>By paper application</u>. Contact the company offering the plan chosen, and ask for an application. Once the application is filled out, mail or fax it back to the company.

    - <u>On the plan's website</u>. Visit the drug plan company's website to see if one can join online.

    - <u>On Medicare's website</u>. One may also be able to join a Medicare drug plan at www.medicare.gov on the web. Select "Compare Medicare Prescription Drug Plans." Not

Chapter 5   **Joining a PDP**
                                                                                                                                   (continued)

all Medicare drug plans offer the option to enroll on the web.

- <u>Over the telephone</u>. One may be able to join by calling the desired plan or by calling 1-800-MEDICARE (1-800-633-4227).

VI. ARE THE COSTS OF PRESCRIPTION DRUGS UNDER PRESCRIPTION DRUG PLANS LESS FOR LOW-INCOME INDIVIDUALS?

Yes.

MMA provides for **subsidies** to meet all or some of the premiums, and cost-sharing payments (deductibles and co-payments) **in the case of certain low-income Medicare beneficiaries with incomes up to one-hundred fifty (150) percent of the Federal poverty level**. Subsidies differ depending on income, Medicaid status and institutional status.

A. Who Are the Low-income Beneficiaries?

These beneficiaries are each a **subsidy-eligible individual** and according to income or status are (i) **full-subsidy-eligible individuals (full-benefit dual eligible)**, (ii) individuals treated (**deemed**) as full-subsidy-eligibles, or (iii) **partial-subsidy individuals. These individuals are discussed below:**

1. **A subsidy-eligible individual** is a Part D-eligible individual who (i) is enrolled in or seeking to enroll in a Part D plan; (ii) has an income below one-hundred fifty (150) percent of the Federal poverty level; and (iii) has resources at or below the thresholds set forth below.

There are two groups of subsidy-eligible, low-income individuals. <u>The first group</u> is composed of persons who either:

- are enrolled in a prescription drug plan;
- have incomes below one-hundred thirty-five (135) percent of Federal poverty level;
- have resources in 2008 below $6,290 for an individual and $9,440 for a couple (increased in future years by the percentage increase in the consumer price index (CPI);

or

are full-benefit dual eligibles without regard to income resources and without regard as to whether they meet other eligibility standards.

<u>The second group</u> of subsidy-eligible individuals is persons meeting the same requirements as above, except that the income level is above one-hundred thirty-five (135) percent but below one-hundred

Chapter 5

Subsidy Programs (continued)

fifty (150) percent of the Federal poverty level and an alternative resource standard is used. The alternative standard in 2008 is $10,490 for an individual and $20,970 for a couple (increased in future years by the percentage increase in the CPI).

2. **A full-subsidy-eligible individual** has full Medicaid status (**full-benefit dual eligible**), income below one-hundred thirty-five (135) percent of the Federal poverty level, resources of less than $6,290 (single person) or less than $9,440 (married couple).

3. **Individuals treated (deemed) as full-subsidy-eligible individuals** are recipients of Supplemental Security Income without Medicaid **or** individuals enrolled in one of the following Medicare savings programs (also called buy-in programs):

- Qualified Medicare beneficiary (QMB);
- Specified low-income Medicare beneficiary (SLMB); or
- Qualifying individual (QI-1) under a state's plan.

4. **Partial-subsidy-eligible individuals** (non-deemed) have (i) income above one-hundred thirty-five (135) percent of the Federal poverty level, but income less that one-hundred fifty (150) percent of the Federal poverty level and (ii) resources that do not exceed $10,490 (2008) if single, or $20,970 if married.

B. **What Part D Drug Subsidies Are Provided to Low-income Individuals?**

The following subsidies are provided to full-subsidy individuals (full-benefit dual eligibles), individuals deemed to be full-benefit dual eligibles, and partial-subsidy individuals:

1. **Full-subsidy-eligible individuals**. The cost-sharing benefits for these eligible Medicaid recipients include the following:

- No premiums;
- No deductible;
- No "donut hole" (the amount of out-of-pocket drug costs that standard benefit beneficiaries are required to pay once their initial coverage limit of $2,510 (2008) is reached);

- $1.05 co-payment for generic drugs, $3.10 for brand-name drugs, up to the out-of-pocket threshold of $4,050 (2008);

2. **"Deemed" full-subsidy-eligible individuals** (Medicare beneficiaries who are "deemed" to be full-benefit dual eligibles).

   The cost-sharing benefits of these individuals include the following:

   - No premiums;
   - No deductible;
   - No donut hole;
   - Co-payment of $2.25 for generic drugs and $5.60 for brand-name drugs, up to the out-of-pocket threshold of $4,050 (2008).

3. **Partial-subsidy eligibles.** The cost-sharing benefits of these individuals are as follows:

   a. Medicare beneficiaries, who are not eligible for Medicaid, with <u>resources less than $10,490 (for a single person) or less than $20,970 (for a married couple) and income below one-hundred thirty-five (135) percent of the Federal poverty level.</u>

   - No premiums;
   - No deductible;
   - Co-payments of $2.25 for each generic drug and $5.60 for each brand-name drug, once the $4,050 (2008) out-of-pocket limit is reached;

   b. Medicare beneficiaries with <u>resources below $10,490 (for a single individual) or $20,970 (for a married couple), and income between one-hundred thirty-five (135) percent and one-hundred fifty (150) percent of the Federal poverty level:</u>

   The **cost-sharing** benefits of these individuals include the following:

   - A sliding scale monthly premium, namely:

Chapter 5   **Subsidy Programs**
                                                                                                                                               (continued)

       - A premium subsidy equal to seventy-five (75) percent of the premium subsidy for individuals with <u>income greater than one-hundred thirty-five (135) percent but at or below one-hundred forty (140) percent of the Federal poverty level.</u>

       - A premium subsidy equal to fifty (50) percent of the premium subsidy standard for individuals with <u>income greater than one-hundred forty (140) percent but at or below one-hundred forty-five (145) percent of the Federal poverty level.</u>

       - A premium subsidy equal to twenty-five (25) percent of the premium for individuals with income greater than one-hundred forty-five (145) percent but below one-hundred fifty (150) percent of the Federal poverty level.

- A $56 deductible;

- Coinsurance of fifteen (15) percent after the deductible, up to the out-of-pocket threshold of $4,050 (2008); and

- Co-payments of $2.25 for each generic drug or $5.60 for each brand-name drug, once the out-of-pocket limit of $4,050 (2008) is reached.

Note: There is no cost-sharing for eligible individuals residing in a medical facility. A "medical facility" is defined as a nursing home, psychiatric center, residential treatment center, developmental center, intermediate care facility. Individuals living in other group residences such as assisted living programs, group homes and adult homes are subject to co-payments.

Chapter 6

CHAPTER 6

MEDICARE ADVANTAGE PLANS (MAP)
A FEDERAL SOURCE OF PAYMENT

I.   WHAT ARE MEDICARE ADVANTAGE PLANS?

All Medicare beneficiaries have the option to receive Medicare benefits through **health plans of private companies**. The plans are part of a program called Part C and are termed Medicare Advantage plans (MAP). <u>The plans are alternatives to Original Medicare fee-for-service</u> (Traditional Medicare). They provide enrollees in the plan with Part A (Hospital) and Part B (Medical) Medicare coverage, and in addition extra benefits (which include the Medicare Part D program covering outpatient prescription drugs (see Chapter 7), and may include vision, hearing, dental and other health services).

All Medicare eligibles entitled to Medicare Part A and enrolled under Medicare Part B, except: (i) individuals with end-stage renal disease, may elect to receive basic Part A/B Medicare benefits through the Original Medicare programs or through Medicare Advantage plans and (ii) an individual who is a Qualified Medicare Beneficiary, a Qualified Disabled and Working Individual, a Specified Low-income Medicare Beneficiary, or otherwise eligible for Medicare and entitled to Medicare cost-sharing under state Medicaid programs.

All Medicare-eligibles are given the **continuing opportunity to switch** among the MAPs or to the Original Medicare plan **during an annual election period** (November and December).

MAPs often have networks and may or may not require enrollees to seek physicians who belong to the plan network or go to a certain hospital to obtain services. Medicare Advantage plans account for nearly nine (9) million of the forty-three (43) million Medicare beneficiaries – one in five of all Medicare enrollees.

Should an individual decide to join a MAP instead of the Original Medicare, he/she:[*]

   – Still is in the Medicare program.

---

[*] This information is supplied by CMS in its handbook *Medicare and You 2007*.

Chapter 6   **Introduction to MAPs**
                                                                                        (continued)

- Still has Medicare rights and protections.
- Still gets complete Medicare Part A and Part B coverage.

    However, the plan may offer different co-payments and deductibles under Parts A and B as long as the premium and cost-sharing are actually equivalent to cost-sharing under Original Medicare.

- Usually gets prescription drug coverage (Part D) through the MAP (see section K below). In most Medicare Advantage plans, if the plan offers Medicare prescription drug coverage and the individual wants drug coverage, he/she must get it from the MAP. In these cases, if an individual joins a stand-alone Medicare prescription drug plan (PDP), he/she will be disenrolled from the MAP. MA sponsors other than MSA and a private fee-for-service (PFFS) plan are required to offer Part D coverage.

- If an individual has a Medicare PFFS plan (one of the MAPs) that does not offer Medicare prescription drug coverage, or if he/she has a Medicare Medical Savings Account Plan (one of the MAPs), he/she can also join a stand-alone Medicare PDP.

- May be able to get extra benefits offered by the plan, such as coverage for vision, hearing, dental, and/or health and wellness programs.

- Must pay the Part B premium.

- Usually will have to pay some other costs (such as co-payments or coinsurance) for the services obtained. <u>Out-of-pocket costs in these plans are generally lower than in the Original Medicare plan, but vary by the services used.</u>

- Will fill the "gaps" in Original Medicare coverage, generally covered by a Medigap policy (Medicare Supplemental Insurance), without the necessity of buying such policy.

- Can get information from Medicare by visiting www.medicare.gov or calling 1-800-MEDICARE (1-800-633-4227).

II. WHAT FEATURES ARE COMMON TO MEDICARE ADVANTAGE PLANS?

Medicare Advantage-eligibles are beneficiaries who are entitled to the benefits of Medicare Part A, are enrolled in Medicare Part B, and do not have end-stage renal disease. They are eligible to enroll in a MAP that serves the geographic area in which they reside. A Part B-enrollee who is not entitled to Part A benefits is ineligible.

All Medicare beneficiaries must choose either Original (Traditional) Medicare or a MAP. Newly eligible enrollees who do not choose a plan are deemed to have chosen the Original Medicare program. Enrollees remain enrolled in a plan of choice until they choose another plan.

The salient characteristics of the Medicare Advantage program are set forth below.

A. What Are the Types of Medicare Advantage Plans?

MAPs may take the following forms:

- **Coordinated Care Plans**. These include (i) **health maintenance organizations** (HMOs) with or without point of service options (POS); (ii) **provider-sponsored organizations** (PSO); (iii) **local and regional preferred provider organizations**; (iv) **religious fraternal benefit organizations**; and (v) **special needs organizations**.

- **Medical Savings Accounts (MSA)**. These are a combination of a high-deductible Medicare Advantage insurance plan and a contribution by Medicare to a Medicare plan.

- **Private Fee-for-Service (PFFS) Plans**. These reimburse hospitals, physicians and other care providers at a rate determined by the plan on a fee-for-service basis without placing the providers at financial risk.

While there is a broad similarity among the plans, certain distinctive and significant differences exist between Coordinated Care Plans on the one hand, and PFFS and MSA plans on the other. For example, unlike Coordinated Care Plans, **PFFS and MSA** plans:

- May impose additional premiums above those established for Medicare basic benefits (i.e., Part A and

Part B services). Hence, enrollees in these plans are subject to payment of unlimited premiums charged by the plans for basic benefits.

- <u>Have no limits on balance billing</u> by physicians not under contract. Hence, a beneficiary may be charged by the non-contract physician any amount above a plan's payment schedule for services rendered.

- <u>Have no requirement for external review</u>, unless a utilization review program is established by the plan.

B.   Do MAPs Have a Minimum Enrollment Requirement?

All plans are required to have <u>a minimum enrollment of five thousand (5,000)</u> in urban areas, <u>or fifteen-hundred (1,500)</u> in rural area, <u>except in the case of PSOs</u> when the minimum standard is fifteen-hundred (1,500) (urban) and five-hundred (500) (rural). The foregoing size requirements may be waived by CMS for up to three (3) years for new plans.

C.   How Does a Beneficiary Enroll or Disenroll in a MAP?

<u>Beneficiaries may enroll or disenroll in a plan by filing an appropriate form with a Medicare Advantage organization</u>. A beneficiary's choice of Medicare coverage, whether Original Medicare or a Medicare Advantage plan, continues until the beneficiary **changes** his/her election, the MAP is discontinued, or the MAP no longer serves the geographic area where the beneficiary resides.

A newly eligible Medicare beneficiary will receive a notice thirty (30) days before the beginning of the initial Medicare Advantage enrollment period. Each November, in conjunction with the annual election period, a publicity campaign is conducted. At least fifteen (15) days before the annual election period that occurs each November, HHS will mail to each Medicare Advantage-eligible individual a notice that explains the coverage options and how to elect a plan.

D.   What Are the Enrollment Periods?

The periods during which elections may be made by individuals are set forth below:

Chapter 6 Features Common to MAPs
(continued)

- **Initial Enrollment**

    Upon attaining eligibility for Medicare, individuals will have a choice between Original Medicare and any Medicare Advantage plan available in their area. Any individual failing to make an election will be deemed to have chosen Original Medicare. This **initial coverage election period** is the period during which the new Medicare-eligible may make an initial election; it begins three (3) months prior to the month he/she is first entitled to both Part A and enrolls in Part B, and ends the last day of the month preceding the month of entitlement.

    An individual who enrolls in a Medicare Advantage plan upon first becoming eligible at age 65 may at any time in the first year of coverage disenroll from the Medicare Advantage plan and enroll in Original Medicare.

- **Open Enrollment and Disenrollment Period**

    There is an annual enrollment/disenrollment election process when beneficiaries are limited to one **change of election during the first three (3) months of the applicable year**. An election made during an open enrollment will become effective on the first day of the first month after the election is made. The foregoing limitations do not apply to changes in election made during an annual coordinated election period or during a special election period.

    A Medicare Advantage organization must accept, without restrictions, waiting period, or pre-existing medical exclusion, all eligible beneficiaries who elect that organization's plan during the initial coverage election period, annual coordinated election period, or under the circumstances described in special election periods below.

- **Annual Coordinated Election Period**

    During this period, all Medicare beneficiaries are free to elect among all available options, including Original Medicare, MA plans, MA-prescription drug plans (MA-PDP), or prescription drug plans (PDPs). The period November 15 through December 31 is considered the annual coordinated election period. Enrollment is effective the following January.

- **Special Election Periods (SEP).**

    An individual may disenroll from a Medicare Advantage plan, and may make a new choice of plans in the SEP in the following events:

    (a) In cases of termination or discontinuance of an organization, the SEP begins when the organization is required to give notice to beneficiaries and ends three (3) months after the notification.

    (b) For a beneficiary who has moved, the SEP runs for three (3) months starting with the month prior to the permanent move and ending the month after the move. The beneficiary may choose an effective date of up to three (3) months after the month when the Medicare Advantage Plan receives the beneficiary's completed enrollment form, but the effective date may not be prior to the date the beneficiary moved or the date the Medicare Advantage organization received the completed enrollment form.

    (c) In the case of **breach of contract or material misrepresentations** by the organization, the SEP begins once CMS agrees that a violation occurred. The length of the SEP depends on whether the beneficiary immediately elects a new Medicare Advantage Plan on disenrollment from the original, or whether the beneficiary first elects Original Medicare before choosing a new Medicare Advantage Plan.

- **Special Enrollment Period for Employees**

    There is a Special Enrollment Period available for individuals who elect their Medicare Advantage Plans through their employers. This special period may be used during the open enrollment period if the employer group health plan is not open for enrollment at the same time as the Medicare Advantage open enrollment; and may also be used when the employer group health plan would permit a beneficiary to change elections based upon personal or life changes. The Special Enrollment Period is only available to Medicare beneficiaries who are members of an employer group health plan that has an arrangement with a Medicare Advantage organization which offers a Medicare Advantage plan to the members of the employer group health plan. Beneficiaries will still have the opportunity to participate in the annual elections. The election periods starts November 15 and ends December 31.

- **Special Rules for Enrolling and Disenrolling in a Medical Savings Account**

A beneficiary can elect to enroll in an MSA plan only upon attaining Medicare eligibility or during the annual coordinated election period in November. New enrollees may revoke their election if they do so before December 15 of the year they make the election (i.e., before their MSA coverage begins). Enrollees may disenroll only during an annual coordinated election period or special election period.

E. What Are the Premiums for MAPs?

There are two (2) types of premiums. (i) The **monthly basic premium** covers basic benefits (Part A and Part B) and additional benefits (such as prescription drugs, hearing aids, dental caps, eyeglasses and preventive care) of Medicare Advantage plans. In the case of a PFFS plan, the basic premium is specified in the plan filed with the Secretary of HHS. (ii) The **monthly supplemental premium** is an amount authorized by the Secretary to cover mandatory and/or supplementary benefits, or in the cases of PFFS and MSA plans, the amount specified in the plan filed with the Secretary.

Except for PFFS and MSA plans, no plan may impose a premium, in addition to the monthly basic premium and monthly supplemental premium authorized by the Secretary of HHS. PFFS and MSA plans may charge unlimited premiums for basic benefits and additional benefits.

Enrollees in all plans financially are required to pay the Medicare Part B premium, which is deducted from their Social Security checks.

F. Are There Limits on Enrollee Cost-sharing?

Yes.

For the basic and additional benefits in Coordinated Care Plans, the monthly basic beneficiary premium (multiplied by 12) and the actuarial value of the cost-sharing (i.e., deductibles, coinsurance and co-payments) applicable to enrollees of a Coordinated Care Plan may not exceed what the actuarial value of an enrollee's cost-sharing would be if he/she were not enrolled in the Coordinated Care Plan.

For PFFS plans, enrollees' cost-sharing with respect to basic and additional benefits may not exceed the actuarial value of the cost-sharing that would apply to enrollees entitled to benefits under Medicare Part A and Part B, if they were not members of the PFFS plan.

Chapter 6   **Features Common to MAPs**
                                                                                                 (continued)

G.   **What Are the Basic, Additional and Supplemental Benefits of MAPs?**

The rules applicable to basic, additional and supplemental benefits, covered by Medicare Advantage plans are set forth below:

- All MAPs must provide coverage for at least the items and services, <u>other than hospice care</u>, for which benefits are available under Original Medicare Parts A and B. These are termed **basic benefits**. In the case of an <u>MSA</u>, such coverage will be provided only after the enrollee meets the annual deductible of the high-deductible health policy that is part of the MSA plan. <u>Coordinated Care Plans</u> may not impose any deductible for basic benefits, but usually require enrollees to pay small **co-payments** to contract providers, (e.g., physicians), as well as for certain additional benefits (e.g., prescription drugs). <u>PFFS</u> plans can impose deductibles, subject to Medicare limits, for Medicare basic services; for **additional benefits** the plans can impose deductibles in an amount they prescribe. Additional benefits are healthcare services not covered by Medicare such as outpatient prescription drugs or waiver of coverage limits (e.g., lifetime limit to reserve days for inpatient hospital care).

- All plans, <u>except PFFS and MSAs</u>, are required to accept Medicare Advantage **capitation** as payment in full for the Medicare basic benefits package.

- All plans, <u>except MSAs</u>, may provide mandatory **supplemental benefits** as part of the overall plan, or **additional benefits** at the option of the beneficiary. <u>MSA</u> plans may not offer supplemental benefits to cover deductibles. **Supplemental benefits** are those not normally covered by Medicare but purchased at the option of the Medicare Advantage enrollee and paid for through a premium or cost-sharing.

- All plans, <u>except a MSA</u>, may provide **supplemental benefits** as part of the overall plan, or **additional**

benefits at the option of the beneficiary. <u>MSA</u> plans may not offer supplemental benefits to cover deductibles.

- A Medicare Advantage <u>PFFS</u> plan may offer **supplemental benefits** to cover some or all of the balance billing amounts, and to cover **additional services** if they are found to be medically necessary.

H. To What Services Does an Enrollee Have Access in Medicare Advantage Coordinated Care Plans and Network MSA Plans?

An enrollee's access to services of Medicare Advantage Coordinated Care Plans and network Medicare Advantage MSA plans are set forth below:

- The plan or organization must maintain a network of appropriate providers.

- <u>A primary care physician</u> (PCP) panel must be established by the organization from which the enrollee may select a PCP. Although CMS does not require it, the organization may require that the enrollee use a PCP. The organization must develop policies regarding methods of coordinating care and must ensure that every enrollee can have a PCP if he or she so chooses. There is no requirement that a treatment plan be updated by a PCP; if a specialist develops a treatment plan, he/she should be the one to update it.

- The organization must ensure it has in effect CMS-approved procedures which identify individuals with complex or serious medical conditions, assess and monitor those conditions and establish a treatment plan which includes an <u>adequate number of direct access visits to specialists</u>.

- The organization must provide or arrange for <u>necessary specialty care</u>. Women enrollees must have the option of direct access to a woman's health specialist within the network for routine and preventive health care. The organization can control the number of direct visits to the specialist, as long as the number is adequate and consistent with the treatment plan.

- <u>Plan services must be made available by the organization 24 hours/day, 7 days/week</u>, when medically necessary.

- The organization must make <u>a best effort attempt to conduct an initial assessment</u> of each enrollee's health needs.

- The organization must cover <u>emergency and urgently needed care</u>. For emergency services obtained outside the organization network, the organization may not charge the enrollee more than $50, or what the organization would charge, whichever is less.

I. How Does Medicare Treat Payments to Medicare Advantage Organizations?

In the traditional fee-for-service Medicare, when another health plan covers benefits for a plan participant who is also a Medicare beneficiary entitled to such benefits under Medicare Part A and/or Part B, Medicare considers that such other plan is the primary payer for benefits and that Medicare is only the secondary payer. Accordingly, should Medicare make payment for the benefits that should have been made by primary payer, Medicare may obtain recovery against the primary payer. A Medicare Advantage organization may take payments from primary payers. Medicare may seek to recover incorrect payments if recovery is sought within three (3) years after services have been rendered.

J. What Emergency Services Must a Medicare Advantage Plan Provide?

Each Medicare Advantage plan must provide for emergency needed services for its enrollees based on a prudent lay person test. The term **"emergency services"** means those inpatient and outpatient services that are furnished by a qualified provider and are needed to evaluate and stabilize an **emergency medical condition**.

The term **"emergency medical condition"** means a medical condition manifesting itself by acute symptoms of sufficient severity, including severe pain, that a prudent lay person who possesses an average knowledge of health and medicine could reasonably expect the absence of immediate medical attention to seriously jeopardize the health of the individual or to cause serious impairment of bodily functions; or serious dysfunctions of a bodily organ part.

For emergency or urgently needed services obtained outside the plan's network, the organization may not charge enrollee more than $50 or what it would charge the enrollee if he/she obtained the service through the MA plan.

K. In Which Instances May a Medicare Advantage Organization Balance Bill or Not?

The following paragraphs detail the instances when Medicare Advantage organizations may balance bill or not.

By Federal law antedating the Balance Budget Act of 1997, the maximum allowable charge (charge limit) is one-hundred fifteen (115) percent of the Medicare-approved charge. The practice of billing up to one-hundred fifteen (115) above the maximum-approved amount is called **balance billing**. A number of states – Connecticut, Massachusetts, Minnesota, New York, Ohio, Pennsylvania, Rhode Island and Vermont – have by state statute partially or completely banned the practice of balance billing. Although the statutes have been challenged in Federal courts on preemption grounds, each has withstood the challenge.

Under the Balanced Budget Act of 1997 which created Medicare+Choice plans (now known as Medicare Advantage plans), health care providers may or may not be permitted to engage in the practice of balance billing – depending upon the type of plan, and whether or not the provider has a contract with the plan.

<u>Under all Medicare Advantage plans, except Medicare Advantage MSA and PFFS plans, non-contracting physicians and other health care providers may not balance bill</u>, but must accept as payment in full from a Medicare Advantage plan enrollee, the amount that would have been paid under Original Medicare. <u>However, a non-contracting physician or other health provider under an MSA or PFFS plan may balance bill without limitation.</u>

Chapter 6   **Features Common to MAPs**
(continued)

L.   **Must a MA Plan Offer Part D Drug Coverage?**

A **Coordinated Care Plan must offer** Part D prescription drug coverage in that plan or in another MA plan in the same area.

A **MSA plan** is not permitted to offer prescription drug coverage, other than that required under Medicare Parts A and B. If a beneficiary enrolls in an MSA plan that does not offer Part D coverage, he/she may also enroll in a prescription drug plan (PDP).

A **private fee-for-service plan** can choose to offer Part D coverage. If a beneficiary enrolls in a PFFS plan, he/she may also enroll in a PDP.

M.   **What Is the Appeal Process for Home Care Denials, Reductions or Termination of Services?**

See **Appendix A** Grievances – Organization Determinations, Reconsiderations and Appeals

See **Appendix B** Fast-track Appeals to the Independent Review Entity (IRE).

APPENDIX A

GRIEVANCES – ORGANIZATION DETERMINATIONS, RECONSIDERATIONS AND APPEALS

Each Medicare Advantage organization must establish internal **grievances procedures**, under which the eligible enrollee, or a provider on behalf of an enrollee, may challenge the denial of coverage or payment for assistance. These grievances procedures are in addition to the **appeals process** discussed below, regarding Organization Determinations, Reconsideration Determinations and Appeals.

The appeals and grievance procedures in Medicare Part C (Medicare Advantage (MA)) plans are different from those applicable to Original Medicare. Reconsideration Determinations are made by the MA organization plans. A Reconsideration Determination by the MA organization is automatically forwarded to the **Independent Review Entity** (IRE) to review the MA organization's reconsideration decision.

1. **GENERAL.**

    Enrollees have the following rights:

    - The right to have **Grievances** between the enrollee and the MA organization heard and resolved (see (2) below).

    - The right to receive a timely **Organization Determination** (see 3(A) below).

    - The right to request an **Expedited Organization Determination** (see 3(A)(c) below).

    - The right to a **Reconsideration** of the adverse Organization Determination by the MA organization (see 3 (B) below).

    - The right to request an **Expedited Reconsideration** (see 3 (B)(c) below).

- If, as a result of a Reconsideration an MA organization affirms, in whole or in part, its adverse organization determination the right to an automatic **Reconsideration Determination made by an Independent Review Entity under contract with CMS** (see 3 (B)(a-c) below).

- The right to an **Administrative Law Judge (ALJ) Hearing** if the amount in controversy is $100 or more (see 3 (C) below).

- The right to request and obtain a **Departmental Appeals Board (DAB) Review** of the ALJ hearing decision (see 3 (D) below).

- The right to **Judicial Review** of the hearing decision if the amount in controversy is $1,000 or more (see 3 (E) below).

2. **GRIEVANCES.**

   (A) <u>**General rule.**</u>

   Each MA organization must provide meaningful procedures for timely hearing and resolving grievances between enrollees and the organization or any other entity or individual through which the organization.

   (B) <u>**Distinguished from appeals.**</u>

   Grievance means any complaint or dispute, other than one that constitutes an Organization Determination, expressing dissatisfaction with any aspect of a MA organization's or provider's operations, activities, or behavior, regardless of whether remedial action is requested.

   Grievance procedures are distinct from appeal procedures, which address Organization Determinations. Upon receiving a complaint, a MA organization must promptly determine whether the complaint is subject to its Appeal or Grievance procedures.

   (C) <u>**Filing Grievance.**</u>

An enrollee must file his grievance with an MA organization, either orally or in writing, within sixty (60) days of the event that gives rise to the grievance.

(D) **Notice of Decision; Time Frame of Decision and Extension.**

The MA organization must notify the enrollee of its decision as expeditiously as the case requires based on the enrollee's health, but no later than thirty (30) days after its receives the grievance. The organization may extend the thirty- (30) day timeframe by up to fourteen (14) days if the enrollee requests the extension or if the organization can demonstrate that the delay is in the best interest of the enrollee. When a MA organization extends the deadline, it must inform the enrollee in writing of the reasons for the delay.

If the enrollee submits the grievance in writing, the MA organization must respond in writing. The organization may respond to oral grievances orally or in writing, unless the enrollee requests a written response. The MA organization must respond to all grievances related quality of care in writing, regardless of how the grievance is filed. The response must include a description of the enrollee's right to file a written complaint with the Quality Improvement Organization (QIO). For any complaint submitted to the QIO, the MA organization must cooperate with the QIO in resolving the complaint.

(E) **Expedited grievances.**

An MA organization must respond to an enrollee's grievance within twenty-four (24) hours if the complaint involves:

-- a MA organization's decision to invoke an extension relating to an Organization Determination or Reconsideration.

-- a MA organization's refusal to grant an enrollee's request for an Expedited Organization Determination or Reconsideration.

An expedited grievance process provides important protections for enrollees who are unable (or prefer not) to obtain a physician's certification that when applying the standard time frame for appeals, would have adverse consequences for the enrollee. By allowing an expedited grievance to proceed under these circumstances, the decision about the grievance would not be the Organization Determination, but rather the plan's appropriate use of its discretion to extend the time frame.

3. **APPEAL PROCESS.**

   (A) <u>**Organization Determinations.**</u>

   Each MA organization must have a procedure for making **timely** Organization Determinations regarding the benefit an enrollee is entitled to receive under a MA plan.

   <u>**An organization determination is any determination made by a MA organization regarding**</u>:

   - Payment for temporary out-of-area renal dialysis services, emergency services, post-stabilization care, or urgently needed services;

   - Payment for any other health services furnished by a provider other than the MA organization that the enrollee believes are covered under Medicare;

   - The MA organization's refusal to provide or pay for services, including the type or level or services, that the enrollee believes should have been furnished, arranged for, or reimbursed by the MA organization;

   - Denial, reduction or termination of a service if the enrollee believes that continuation of the services is medically necessary (see Appendix B, item 1); or

   - Failure of the MA organization to timely furnish or pay for health care services.

   The time frames within which an organization must make its determinations depends upon whether related they are to <u>services</u> or to <u>payment</u>, and are divided into the following two (2) categories – <u>standard</u> (see (a) and (b) below) and <u>expedited</u> (see (c) below).

   (a) <u>Standard Organization Determinations (**service related**)</u>.

When an enrollee or representative requests a service, the organization must notify the enrollee in writing of its determination as expeditiously as the enrollee's health condition requires, but no later than (that is, not to exceed (NTE) fourteen (14) days after the day on which the organization received the enrollee's request for a determination. This time frame is subject to a possible extension requested by the enrollee, or by the organization if there is a justified need for additional information on the part of the organization and the extension is in the interest of the enrollee.

(b) Standard Organization Determinations (**payment related**).

A difference is made in the time frames within which determinations must be made where a claim for payment is (i) a "**clean claim**," and (ii) other claims, for Payment. When there is a request for payment (other than a clean claim), the organization must make a determination NTE sixty (60) days from the date of receipt of the payment request. However, clean claims must be paid NTE thirty (30) days of receiving the payment request. Clean claims are claims that have no defect or impropriety, do not lack any required substantiating documentation, and do not require special treatment that prevents timely payments.

(c) Expedited Organization Determinations (**service related**).

An enrollee or physician (whether affiliated with the organization or not) can orally or in writing request an Expedited Organization Determination with respect to the organization's refusal to provide service (when the enrollee has not received the service outside the plan) or its discontinuance of the service. Requests for determination as to payments are not subject to Expedited Organization Determinations.

If the organization approves the request for an expedited organization determination or if a physician (whether affiliated with the organization or not) requests an expedited time frame, indicating that to apply the standard time frame (i.e., fourteen (14) days) for making the determination could serious jeopardize the life or health of the enrollee, or the enrollee's ability to regain maximum function, then the organization must:

    (i) make its determination, NTE seventy-two (72) hours after receiving the request, (subject to possible extension of time, if the enrollee requests the extension or the organization justifies a need for additional information and that the delay is for the benefit of the enrollee); and

    (ii) first notify the enrollee of the determination orally, and then send written notification within two (2) days of the oral notification.

If the organization denies a request for expedited action, it must give the enrollee oral notice of the denial, and within three (3) days, send a letter explaining that a determination will be made NTE fourteen (14) days of receiving the request, and that the enrollee can file a grievance with the organization, if he/she so desires. If the organization denies a service request, it must so notify the enrollee, and inform the enrollee of his/her right to a Reconsideration Determination and to the rest of the appeal process.

(B) **Reconsideration Determinations.**

This is the first step in the review of an adverse Organization Determination. A request for reconsideration may be made by the enrollee or his/her representative or an assignee of the enrollee, or a legal representative of a deceased enrollee's estate.

The request for reconsideration must be in writing and filed with the organization that made the Organization Determination, or a Social Security office or, in the case of a qualified railroad retirement beneficiary, a Railroad Retirement Benefit office. The request must be made NTE sixty (60) days of the date of the notice of the Organization Determination.

The request may be for a Standard Reconsideration Determination (see (a) and (b) below) or an Expedited Reconsideration Determination (service related) (see (c) below), as set forth below.

(a) Standard Reconsideration Determination (**service related**).

Should the organization make a Reconsideration Determination that is completely favorable to the enrollee, then the organization must issue the determination as expeditiously as the enrollee's health condition requires, and must authorize or provide the service, NTE thirty (30) days from the date of receiving the request for reconsideration.

Should the organization affirm in whole or in part its adverse organization determination (by making a determination that is wholly or partially unfavorable to the enrollee), the case file and the issues that remain in **dispute must be sent to, and reviewed and resolved by an Independent Review Entity (IRE)** selected by the CMS. This submission must be made as expeditiously as the enrollee's condition requires, but not after more than thirty (30) days, (subject to extension), from the date of the request for review by the IRE.

When the IRE makes its determination, it must mail notice of this determination to the parties and to the CMS not later than thirty (30) days from the date of the request for IRE review. If the IRE determination is adverse, the enrollee must be informed of his/her right to an ALJ hearing, if the amount in controversy is $100 or more. However, if the entity should rule in favor of the enrollee, the organization must authorize or provide the service as expeditiously as the enrollee's health requires, but not later (NTE) than sixty (60) days from the date the organization receives notice reversing its organization determination.

(b) Standard Reconsideration Determination (**payment related**).

Should the organization make a reconsideration determination that is completely favorable to the enrollee, the organization must issue its determination and pay the requested payment NTE sixty (60) days from the date it receives the request for reconsideration.

Should the organization make a Reconsideration Determination that is partially or completely unfavorable to the enrollee, **it must send the case file to an IRE**, selected by the CMS, for review and resolution NTE sixty (60) days from the date it receives the reconsideration request for **review and resolution.** The entity must render its decision as expeditiously as an enrollee's health condition requires, but not more than (NTE) thirty (30) days (subject to extension in certain cases) from the date it received the request for IRE review.

The IRE must send the enrollee and the CMS written notice of its determination, stating the reasons for its determination. Should the entity's decision be adverse to the enrollee, the notice must inform the enrollee of his/her right to an ALJ hearing, if the amount in controversy is $100 or more.

Should the entity decide in favor of the enrollee, the organization must pay for the service as expeditiously as the enrollee' health condition requires, but not more than (NTE) sixty (60) calendar days from the date the organization receives notice reversing the organization determination.

(c) Expedited Reconsideration Determination (**service related**).

Enrollees, their representatives, or physicians may request an expedited Reconsideration of an Organization Determination involving a request relating to a service, or discontinuance of a service. **Expedited Reconsiderations may not involve a payment related case.**

The organization can first notify the enrollee orally, but must send a written notice NTE two (2) days.

If the organization makes an Expedited Reconsideration, which is completely favorable to the enrollee, it must issue such determination as expeditiously as the enrollee's health condition requires, but not more than seventy-two (72) hours after receiving the request. If the organization does issue such an Expedited Reconsideration (i.e., one which is completely favorable to the enrollee), the organization must authorize or provide the service as expeditiously as the enrollee's health condition requires, but not later than thirty (30) days from the date the organization received the reconsideration request.

The organization may deny an enrollees request for expedited reconsideration but must grant the request of any physician for an Expedited Reconsideration.

If an organization denies the request for an Expedited Reconsideration, it must give the enrollee prompt oral notice and follow up, NTE three (3) days with a written notice that (i) the request was denied and (ii) the Reconsideration Determination will be made by the organization in the standard time frame for reconsiderations (see 1(a)) NTE thirty (30) days of receiving the request.

If the organization makes an Expedited Reconsideration that is partially or wholly unfavorable to the enrollee, **it must deliver the case file to the IRE** as expeditiously as the enrollee's health condition requires, but not later than (NTE) twenty-four (24) hours of its determination. The IRE must make its decision as expeditiously as the enrollee's condition requires, but not later (NTE) than seventy-two (72) hours (subject to a possible extension in certain cases). The entity must mail a written notice of its determination to the enrollee, and to the CMS, stating the reasons for its decision. If the decision is adverse to the enrollee, the notice must notify the enrollee of his/her right to a hearing before the ALJ, if the amount in controversy is $100 or more.

If the entity should decide in favor of the enrollee, the Organization must authorize or provide the requested Service as expeditiously as the enrollee's health requires, but not later than seventy-two (72) hours from the date the organization receives notice reversing its organization determination.

(C) Hearing before ALJ.

If the amount in controversy is $100 or more, the enrollee (or other proper party acting on his/her behalf), if dissatisfied with the IRE determination, has a right to a hearing before an Administrative Law Judge (ALJ). The written request for a hearing is made before either the organization that issued the organization determination, an Social Security office or, in the case of a qualified railroad retirement beneficiary, an Railroad Retirement Benefit office, whereupon the aforesaid organization must forward the request to the IRE that made the IRE determination, and the entity must transfer the case to the appropriate ALJ hearing office. The enrollee must file his/her request for a hearing NTE sixty (60) days of the date of the determination by the IRE.

(D) Departmental Appeals Board Review.

If the enrollee (or any proper party to the hearing) is dissatisfied with the ALJ hearing decision, he/she may request the Departmental Appeals Board to review the decision.

(E) Judicial Review.

Any party, including the organization, may request judicial review of an ALJ final decision, if the amount in controversy is $1,000 or more.

APPENDIX B

FAST-TRACK APPEALS TO
THE INDEPENDENT REVIEW ENTITY

The Secretary of HHS has contracted with Qualified Improvement Organizations (QIO) as the Independent Review Entity to review and affirm the **termination** of services. An enrollee has the right to a fast-track appeal to the IRE of such denial. The steps of the appeal process are set forth below.

1. **Issuance of notice.**

    Prior to any termination of service, the provider (i.e., home health agency, skilled nursing facility and comprehensive outpatient rehabilitation facility) must deliver advance written notice to an enrollee of the MA organization's decision to terminate service. The notice must be provided no later than two days before the proposed end of services.

2. **Content of notice.**

    The notice must state: the date that coverage ends; a description of the enrollee's right to a fast-track appeal to the IRE; and the availability of other MA appeal procedures.

3. **Effectiveness of notice.**

    To be effective, the notice must be dated and signed by the enrollee evidencing receipt.

    The MA organization is required to pay for continued services until two (2) days after the enrollee receives the notice.

4. **Right to fast-track appeal to an IRE.**

    An enrollee of an MA organization has a right to a fast-track appeal to the IRE of a MA organization's decision to terminate provider services. This can be requested of the IRE in writing or by telephone by noon of the first day after the day of delivery of the termination notice. If an enrollee fails to make a timely request to the IRE, he/she may resort to the standard appeal process.

5. Continuation of coverage.

Coverage of provider services continues to the date and time designated in a termination notice, unless an enrollee appeals and the IRE reverses the MA organization's decision.

6. Actions by IRE.

Upon receipt of enrollee's request for an appeal, the IRE must immediately notify the MA organization and the provider of the appeal request. The IRE must make a decision and notify the enrollee, the MA organization, and the provider of its decision, by close of business of the day after it receives the information it requires. The IRE can defer its decision until it receives the necessary information from the MA. Coverage continues until the IRE makes its decision.

7. Reconsiderations of IRE decisions.

An enrollee may request reconsideration by the IRE within sixty (60) days after notification that the IRE has upheld the decision. The reconsideration must be rendered expeditiously, but no later than within fourteen (14) days of receipt of the enrollee's request. If affirmed in whole or part, the enrollee may successively appeal to the ALJ, the DAB and a Federal court.

Chapter 6

III. WHAT SPECIAL FEATURES DO THE DIFFERENT MEDICARE ADVANTAGE PLANS HAVE?

Set forth below is a list of the appendices which describe the **special features**[*] explained in the plan specified:

Appendix C Coordinated Care Plans (CCP)

- Appendix C-1 HMO Plans
- Appendix C-2 Preferred Provider Organization (PPO) Plans
- Appendix C-3 Provider-sponsored Organization (PSO)
- Appendix C-4 Religious Fraternal Benefits (RFB) Plans
- Appendix C-5 Specialized Medicare Advantage Plans for Special Needs Beneficiaries (SNP)

Appendix D Medical Savings Account (MSA) Plans

Appendix E Private Fee-for-Service (PFFS) Plans

---

[*] These appendices may repeat some of the same information about special features found in section II above.

Appendix C

COORDINATED CARE PLANS (CCP)

The various Medicare Advantage (MA) plans are classified into three (3) general types: Coordinated Care Plans (CCP), Medical Saving Account (MSA) plans, and Private Fee-for-Service (PFFS) plans.

The specifications set forth below apply to <u>Coordinated Care Plans</u>.

1. **<u>Definition.</u>**

   An MA CCP is offered by an MA organization that <u>includes a network</u> of providers that are under contract or arrangement with the organization to deliver at least the benefit package authorized by CMS. The network of providers must be approved by CMS to ensure that all applicable requirements are met, including access and availability standards, service area requirements, and quality standards.

2. **<u>Provider Network.</u>**

   The organization must maintain a network of appropriate providers.

3. **<u>Primary Care Physician Panel.</u>**

   <u>A **panel of primary care physicians** (PCP) must be established by the organization from which the enrollee may select a PCP</u>. If an enrollee desires to change his/her PCP, the enrollee can ask the plan for the names of the other plan doctors in the plan area. There is no requirement that a treatment plan be updated by a PCP; any health professional or team of health professionals may develop the treatment plan. If a specialist develops a treatment plan, he/she should be the one to update it.

4. **<u>Serious Medical Conditions.</u>**

   The organization must ensure it has in effect CMS-<u>approved procedures</u> which (i) <u>identify individuals with complex or serious medical conditions</u>; (ii) <u>assess and monitor</u> those conditions; and (iii) <u>establish a treatment plan</u> which includes an adequate number of direct access visits to specialist.

5. **Specialty Care.**

The organization must provide or arrange for necessary specialty care and, in particular for women enrollees, the option of direct access to a women's health specialist within the network for routine and prevention health care services. The CMS regulations do not prohibit the organization limiting the number of direct visits to the specialist, as long as the number is adequate and consistent with the treatment plan. Enrollees in CCP plans, **other than HMOs or PSOs,** do not need a referral to a specialist.

6. **Hours of Operation.**

Plan services must be made available by the organization 24 hours a day, 7 days a week, when medically necessary.

7. **Initial Assessment.**

The organization must make a "best effort" attempt to conduct an initial assessment of each enrollee's health needs.

8. **Premiums.**

Enrollees are required to pay only the monetary basic premiums, and supplemental premium authorized by the CMS.

9. **Charge Limits (Balance Billing).**

a. **When a provider does not have a contract with the plan**. A physician or other provider who does not have a contract establishing payment amounts for services furnished to an enrollee in one of the Coordinated Care Plan organizations is required to accept as payment in full for covered services amounts that physicians or other providers could collect if the individual were not enrolled in such organization (i.e., the amount that Original Medicare fee-for-services would have paid to an enrollee, if enrolled in Original Medicare).

b. **When a provider does have a contract with the plan**. A physician or other provider of services who has a contract with the plan establishing payment amounts for services furnished to an enrollee of a Coordinated Care Plan organization is required to accept as payment in full for covered services the amount set forth in the plan's fee schedule.

10. **Flexibility of Choice by a Medicare-eligible Among Coordinated Care Plans.**

A Medicare-eligible may choose from among a variety of CCPs. They include, but are not limited to: Health Maintenance Organization (HMO) plans (with or without point-of-service options), plans offered by local and/or regional Preferred Provider Organization (PPO) plans, Provider-sponsored Organization (PSO) plans, Religious Fraternal Benefits (RFB) plans, and Specialized MA plans for Special Needs Beneficiaries (SNP).

11. **State Licensure and Other State Requirements.**

Except in the case of a PSO (granted a waiver of state licensing requirements), all organizations offering the CCP must meet the state licensure requirements. Thus, the CCP must be offered by an entity that is (i) appropriately licensed as a risk-bearing entity by the state, and (ii) eligible to offer health insurance or health benefit coverage, in each state in which it offers an MA plan. The coverage which the entity provides may be on an indemnity basis, as in the case of PPO, or a pre-capitated basis, as in the case of an HMO. To offer a CCP, the entity does not need to be licensed specifically as an HMO, PSO or PPO.

12. **Outpatient Part D Coverage**

All CCPs must offer their enrollees Part D coverage.

APPENDIX C-1

HMO PLANS

A Health Maintenance Organization (HMO) is one of the Coordinated Care plans. The specifications for an HMO are set forth below.

1. **Definition.**

    The HMO is a managed care arrangement between: (i) individual participants and the HMO, which provides to the participants through a network of doctors and other health providers an array of Medicare-covered medical services (physician services, and a range of laboratory, x-ray and ancillary services); and (ii) the HMO and Medicare which pays the HMO a fixed predetermined, periodic fee, known as a **capitation fee**.

2. **Lock-in Feature.**

    The plan participants are **locked-in** to and may only use a network provider (except for emergency or urgent care), unless the HMO has opted for a point of service option for its enrollees (see point 4 below). Services received by a participant, other than through the HMO network, will not be paid for by the HMO; the participant is personally liable for these out-of-network services.

3. **Primary Care Physician – Specialist.**

    An enrollee generally will be asked to choose a **primary care doctor** (commonly referred to as "**gatekeeper**"). Should the enrollee seek a **specialist**, he/she needs a referral from the primary care doctor, except that generally a woman does not need a reference for a yearly screening mammogram, or two in-network pap tests and pelvic exams (at least every other year), provided the specialist is in the network.

4. **Prescription Drugs**

    The HMO must offer enrollees prescription drug coverage. They are not allowed to obtain drug coverage through Part D plans.

5. **Point of Service Option**

    (a) <u>Definition</u>

    A point of service (POS) option is an option that a Medicare Advantage Health Maintenance Organization may offer a Medicare-eligible through a CCP <u>or</u> network Medical Saving Account (MSA) plan (whether operated on a indemnity or prepaid capitated basis) to obtain outside the plan specified health care items and services from providers (non-contract providers) that do not have a contract with the MA organization. The plan with the POS option feature is required to provide, at a minimum, all Medicare-covered services available to beneficiaries under Original Medicare fee-for-service coverage available through Medicare Parts A and B. Should a participant choose care outside of the plan's network, he/she is subject to paying coinsurance, co-payments and deductibles, which are usually higher than in a typical CCP.

    (b) <u>Mandatory Supplemental or Optional Supplemental Benefit</u>

    A CCP may offer a POS option <u>as a mandatory supplemental benefit, or an optional supplemental benefit</u>. **A** network MSA plan may offer the POS option but only as a supplemental benefit**.**

    (c) <u>Cap on Enrollee's Liability</u>

    There <u>must be a plan cap</u> placed by the plan on a beneficiary's total annual financial liability under a POS benefit. The enrollee must be clearly informed about all of the estimated potential costs when enrolling in the plan.

    (d) <u>Direct Access</u>

    A Medicare beneficiary may not use a POS option to seek direct access to a specialist within the plan network. The beneficiary must comply with the rules of the plan typically requiring prior authorization (**pre-certification**) by a primary care physician, or other network health professionals.

APPENDIX C-1

HMO PLANS

A Health Maintenance Organization (HMO) is one of the Coordinated Care plans. The specifications for an HMO are set forth below.

1. **Definition.**

    The HMO is a managed care arrangement between: (i) individual participants and the HMO, which provides to the participants through a network of doctors and other health providers an array of Medicare-covered medical services (physician services, and a range of laboratory, x-ray and ancillary services); and (ii) the HMO and Medicare which pays the HMO a fixed predetermined, periodic fee, known as a **capitation fee**.

2. **Lock-in Feature.**

    The plan participants are **locked-in** to and may only use a network provider (except for emergency or urgent care), unless the HMO has opted for a point of service option for its enrollees (see point 4 below). Services received by a participant, other than through the HMO network, will not be paid for by the HMO; the participant is personally liable for these out-of-network services.

3. **Primary Care Physician – Specialist.**

    An enrollee generally will be asked to choose a **primary care doctor** (commonly referred to as "**gatekeeper**"). Should the enrollee seek a **specialist**, he/she needs a referral from the primary care doctor, except that generally a woman does not need a reference for a yearly screening mammogram, or two in-network pap tests and pelvic exams (at least every other year), provided the specialist is in the network.

4. **Prescription Drugs**

    The HMO must offer enrollees prescription drug coverage. They are not allowed to obtain drug coverage through Part D plans.

5. **Point of Service Option**

   (a) <u>Definition</u>

   A point of service (POS) option is an option that a Medicare Advantage Health Maintenance Organization may offer a Medicare-eligible through a CCP <u>or</u> network Medical Saving Account (MSA) plan (whether operated on a indemnity or prepaid capitated basis) to obtain outside the plan specified health care items and services from providers (non-contract providers) that do not have a contract with the MA organization. The plan with the POS option feature is required to provide, at a minimum, all Medicare-covered services available to beneficiaries under Original Medicare fee-for-service coverage available through Medicare Parts A and B. Should a participant choose care outside of the plan's network, he/she is subject to paying coinsurance, co-payments and deductibles, which are usually higher than in a typical CCP.

   (b) <u>Mandatory Supplemental or Optional Supplemental Benefit</u>

   A CCP may offer a POS option <u>as a mandatory supplemental benefit, or an optional supplemental benefit</u>. **A network MSA plan may offer the POS option but only as a supplemental benefit.**

   (c) <u>Cap on Enrollee's Liability</u>

   There <u>must be a plan cap</u> placed by the plan on a beneficiary's total annual financial liability under a POS benefit. The enrollee must be clearly informed about all of the estimated potential costs when enrolling in the plan.

   (d) <u>Direct Access</u>

   A Medicare beneficiary may not use a POS option to seek direct access to a specialist within the plan network. The beneficiary must comply with the rules of the plan typically requiring prior authorization (**pre-certification**) by a primary care physician, or other network health professionals.

APPENDIX C-2
PREFERRED PROVIDER ORGANIZATION (PPO) PLANS

One specific type of the several MA coordinated care plans is a **Preferred Provider Organization plan**.

1. Definition of PPO.

A PPO plan is an arrangement between an employer or insurance company and network of health care providers whereby the providers, called **preferred providers, have agreed to a contractually specified reimbursement for covered services** with the organization offering the plan. As part of the arrangement, the **insurance company or employer negotiates discounted fees with the PPO** so that the insured enrollees receive lower than the customary fee-for-services basis. A form of managed care, the PPO plan is a variant of the classic HMO; however, PPO **enrollees may visit any doctor in the network without a referral, and choose doctors outside of the provider network**, usually for higher fees and/or deductibles.

2. Licensure by State as a Risk-bearing Entity.

In order for a PPO to offer a MA plan as a separate entity all unto itself, it is **required to be licensed by the state** as a **risk-bearing** entity. However, if a PPO is not so licensed, it may enter into partnership or contract with a state-licensed indemnity carrier or state-licensed HMO and "rent" out its PPO network of health care products to that licensee. In such a case, the PPO may operate in conjunction with the licensed carrier or HMO under a PPO plan; and CMS will defer to the applicable licensing state, as to whether the PPO may accept partial capitation from the licensed carrier or HMO.

3. Limit of Enrollee's Liability.

An entity offering a PPO plan must limit an enrollee's financial liability to providers under a PPO plan in the same manner that liability is limited under an HMO plan or any other type of CCP. That is, the sum of the premium for basic benefits and the actuarial value of all out-of-pocket expenses for such benefits (including the actuarial value of cost-sharing for nonparticipating providers of the PPO) cannot exceed the actuarial value of deductibles and coinsurance for Original Medicare fee-for-services.

4. Prescription Drugs

PPOs must offer enrollees prescription drug coverage. Enrollees do not have the option of obtaining other Part D plans.

5. Local and Regional Plans - Definitions.

Commencing January 1, 2006, the single type of PPO in the definition of CCP was expanded into two – "local" and "regional" Coordinated plans. Regional plans are subject to several rules different from those of local plans but are structured as PPOs.

(a) **Regional Plans.** A **MA regional plan** is a coordinated care plan, structured as a PPO, that services one or more entire regions. A MA regional plan: (i) has a network of providers that have agreed to contractually specified reimbursement for covered benefits with the organization offering the plan; (ii) provides reimbursement for all covered benefits regardless of whether such benefits are provided within such network of providers; and (iii) has a service area that spans one or more entire MA regions.

Regional PPOs can only be offered in an MA region, which is defined as an area within the fifty (50) states and the District of Columbia. Congress did not include Puerto Rico or the other U.S. territories in the areas in which organizations could offer regional PPOs.

Regional plans are subject to several different rules than MA local plans, but are structured as PPOs. While local PPO plans may choose the counties in which they wish to operate as Medicare Advantage plans, regional plans must cover an entire region.

(b) **Local Plans.** An MA local plan is an MA plan that is not an MA regional plan. Under current law, MA local plans service county or equivalent areas as specified by the Secretary of HHS.

6. Moratorium on Formation and Expansion of Local PPOs.

In the first two (2) years of formation of regional plans, a moratorium was imposed on the formation or expansion of local plans that operate as PPOs. Starting in 2006, only local PPO plans in the current demonstration areas are authorized. Accordingly, an MA organization cannot offer a new PPO plan in a service area if the MA organization did not offer a PPO plan in that service area in 2005. The MA organization must have actually enrolled beneficiaries into the plan prior to January 1, 2006. The CMS determines the boundaries for the regions in which regional plans operate.

CMS shared risk with MA regional plans during 2006 and 2007. This was intended to encourage plans to enter the regional market and to provide assistance to plans during the start-up phase under the new MA program.

7. Single Deductible Out-of-Pocket Limit of Regional Plans.

MA regional plans have a single deductible for both Part A and Part B benefits. The single deductible may be applied differentially for in-network services and waived for preventive or other items and services.

8. Catastrophic Limits of Regional Plans.

MA regional plans are required to have a **catastrophic limit** on beneficiary out-of-pocket expenditures for in-network benefits under the Original Medicare program. Similarly, MA Regional plans must provide a **total catastrophic limit** on beneficiary out-of-pocket expenditures for in- and out-of-network benefits under the Original Medicare program. The total out-of-pocket catastrophic limit may be higher than the in-network catastrophic limit, but may not increase the limit applicable to in-network services. MA plans must track the deductible and catastrophic limits based on incurred, rather than paid, out-of-pocket beneficiary costs, and notify beneficiaries and providers when the limit has been reached.

9. **State Licenses – Regional Plans.**

CMS may temporarily waive state license requirements in order to facilitate the offering of Regional MA plans in regions encompassing multiple states. However, MA plans will need to be licensed by at least one state in the region and are required to have submitted applications in all of the other states. In addition, the licensure waiver is temporary, and in most cases CMS expects the waiver to be for less than a year.

Appendix C-3
PROVIDER-SPONSORED ORGANIZATION (PSO) PLANS

The PSO is one specific type of the several alternative coordinated care plans.

1. **Overview.**

    A variety of health care providers, such as physicians and hospitals, may integrate themselves into a provider-sponsored network organization, and through that organization create and administer a managed care plan that provides a wide spectrum of medical services to patients. **Unlike other coordinated care plans**, a PSO directly enrolls individuals, and no insurance carrier participates in the arrangement.

2. **Definition.**

    A PSO is a public or private entity:

    - that is established or organized under state law and operated by a health care provider or by a group of affiliated health care providers;

    - that provides a substantial proportion of the required services under a contract directly through the provider or group of providers; and

    - where the providers share substantial financial risk with respect to the provision of health services and have at least a majority stake in the entity.

3. **Minimum Number of Enrollees.**

    In order to qualify as a provider for a risk-basis contract, a PSO must have at least fifteen-hundred (1,500) enrollees in urban areas, or in rural areas five-hundred (500) enrollees.

4. **Risk-bearing Entity.**

Generally, a PSO must be organized under state law as a risk-bearing entity eligible to offer health insurance or health benefits in each state in which it offers a Medicare Advantage plan.

5. **Services to Enrollees.**

The plan is required to provide enrollees, through its physicians and other providers, services not less than those items and services available under Medicare Part A and Part B, <u>other than hospice care</u>.

In order for enrollees to receive coverage for services rendered by a provider outside the PSO, a referral from the enrollee's primary care physician typically is required.

6. **Prescription Drugs.**

PSOs are required to offer their enrollees prescription drug coverage. Enrollees may not obtain other Part D drug coverage.

7. **Payment Limitations (Charge Limits).**

Physicians <u>under contract</u> with the plan may not charge above the plan's fee payments schedule. Physicians <u>not under contract</u> with the plan may not charge for basic benefits more than the total amount payable under Original Medicare.

APPENDIX C-4
RELIGIOUS FRATERNAL BENEFITS (RFB) PLANS

The RFB is one specific type of the several alternative coordinated care plans, including PFFS and MSA plans. The special characteristics of the RFB plan are set forth below:

1. **Definition.**

    A RFB plan is one that:

    - is offered by a religious fraternal benefit society, only to the members of the church, convention, or affiliated group.

    - permits all members to enroll without regard to health status-related factors.

    - must be offered by a religious fraternal benefit society that:

        a) is described under §501(c) (8) of the Internal Revenue Code and is exempt from taxation under §501(a) of that enactment;

        b) is affiliated with, carries out the tenets of, and shares a religious bond with, a church or convention or association of churches or an affiliated group of churches;

        c) offers, in addition to the MA Religious Fraternal Benefits Society plan, at least the same level of health coverage to individuals not entitled to Medicare benefits, who are members of such church, convention or group; and

        d) does not impose any limitation on membership in the society based on any health status-related factors.

Appendix C-4 - Religious Fraternal Benefits Plans (continued)

2. **State License.**

As with other types of coordinated care plans, an entity offering an RFB plan must be organized and licensed under the state law as a risk-bearing entity eligible to offer health insurance or health benefits coverage in each state in which it offers an MA plan. The RFB must meet all other of the state's licensing requirements.

3. **Network of Health Professionals Is Required.**

An organization offering an RFB plan must do more than merely pay health care claims on behalf of its beneficiaries. The plan must meet the definition of a coordinated care plan. As such, the organization must have a network of health professionals and meet the applicable access, availability, service area and quality assurance requirements of a coordinated care plan.

4. **Enrollees May Be Limited to Members of the Church.**

RFP plans have a major distinguishing factor from other types of coordinated care plans. They are allowed to limit enrollment to members of the church. A religious fraternal benefit society offering an MA plan may restrict the enrollment of individuals in the plan to individuals who are members of the church, convention, or group with which the society is affiliated.

5. **Primary Doctors – Specialists.**

Enrollees are not limited to service of primary doctors or specialists in the network and may choose a doctor (including a specialist) outside of the network, but often for higher fees and deductibles.

6. **Prescription Drugs.**

RFBs are required to offer their enrollees prescription drug coverage. Enrollees may not obtain other Part D drug coverage.

APPENDIX C-5
SPECIALIZED MEDICARE ADVANTAGE PLANS FOR SPECIAL NEEDS BENEFICIARIES (SNP)

The Special Needs Plan (SNP) is one specific type of the several MA Coordinated Care plans.

1. **Defined.**

   Commencing January 1, 2006, **MMA authorized SNPs as coordinated care plans** that exclusively or "disproportionately" serve special needs individuals and provide Part D benefits to all enrollees. CMS has designated these plans as meeting the requirements of a SNP, as determined on a case-by-case basis. The establishment of SNPs allows MAPs that have targeted clinical programs for special needs individuals to enroll them exclusively.

   (a) CMS has defined a **disproportionate** percentage SNP as one that enrolls a greater proportion of the target group of special needs individuals than occurs nationally in the Medicare population based on data acceptable to CMS.

   (b) A **special needs individual** means an MA-eligible individual who is institutionalized, is entitled to medical assistance under a state plan, under Title XIX of the Social Security Act, or has a severe or disabling chronic condition and would benefit from enrollment in a specialized MA plan. For the purposes of special needs individuals, **institutionalized** means continuously residing or being expected to continuously reside for ninety (90) days or longer in a long-term care facility that is a skilled nursing facility (SNF), nursing facility (NF), SNF/NF, an intermediate care facility for the mentally retarded, or an inpatient psychiatric facility. CMS may also consider as institutionalized those individuals living in the community but requiring a level of care equivalent to that of those individuals living in those long-term care facilities.

2. **Eligibility.**

To be eligible to elect a Special Needs plan, the beneficiary must:

- meet the definition of a special needs individual,
- meet the eligibility requirements for that specific SNP, and
- be eligible to elect an MA plan.

CMS may exclude beneficiaries with ESRD from eligibility. It also has the authority to designate certain MA plans as SNPs if they disproportionately serve special needs beneficiaries. Furthermore, the SNPs may restrict eligibility solely to those individuals who are in one or more classes of special needs individuals.

A beneficiary enrolled in a SNP who no longer meets the eligibility criteria has **continued eligibility** for a SNP if he/she can reasonably be expected to meet the criteria of the plan within a six- (6) month period. In such a case, the enrollee is deemed to continue to be eligible for the MA plan for a period of not less than thirty (30) days but not to exceed six (6) months. The MA organization may choose any length of time from thirty (30) days to six (6) months for deemed continued eligibility as long as it applies this period consistently among all members in its plan and fully informs its members of the time period.

Beneficiaries already enrolled in an MA plan that CMS later designates as an SNP may not be involuntarily disenrolled because they do not meet the definition of special needs individuals. They may continue to be enrolled in the plan or choose to elect another MA plan during the appropriate election periods provided to all MA eligible beneficiaries.

Grandfathered SNP beneficiaries are distinguished from beneficiaries who join a new SNP and then lose their special needs status on other than a temporary basis. Those special needs beneficiaries would be involuntarily disenrolled after losing their special needs status (and after any period of deemed continued eligibility, if appropriate, as explained above) and receiving proper notice.

Chapter 6

Appendix C-5 Special Needs Plans
(continued)

3. **Bidding Methodology.**

   SNPs have to prepare and submit bids like other MA plans.

4. **Payments to SNPs.**

   SNPs are paid the same as other MA plans, based on the plan's enrollment. There are no special payment features specific to special needs plans. However, a **risk adjustment payment methodology** is being phased in for all MA plans. Under risk adjustment, payments are more accurate because they reflect the health status of an organization's enrollees. Therefore, to the extent that a SNP enrolls less healthy beneficiaries, it will receive higher payments to account for higher risk health status.

5. **Prescription Drugs.**

   SNPs <u>must</u> provide prescription drug Part D coverage. Enrollees are not allowed to obtain other Part D drug coverage.

APPENDIX D
MEDICAL SAVINGS ACCOUNT (MSA) PLANS

1. **Background**

<u>Private</u> MSAs, established by employers for some time, have enabled employees to obtain and pay for high-deductible catastrophic health insurance polices. The private MSA, still in effect, has stimulated development of two <u>Federal</u> demonstration projects. <u>The first of these projects was authorized in 1996 under the Health Insurance Portability and Accountability Act (HIPAA)</u>. It created a four- (4) year pilot MSA program which, effective January 1, 1997, allowed a maximum of 750,000 Medicare beneficiaries to be covered by a high-deductible catastrophic health insurance policy, and to receive certain favorable tax treatment. <u>The Balanced Budget Act of 1997 created a second Federal demonstration project</u> called Medical Savings Account (MSA) Plan. Enrollment was available to a maximum cap of 390,000 Medicare beneficiaries. **Under MMA, MA organizations are <u>now authorized</u> to offer MSA plans as a permanent option; <u>the enrollment cap was eliminated</u>**. MSA plans are considered "local" plans.

2. **Eligibility.**

   (a) Individuals, subject to the limitations mentioned in items (2)-(4) below, who are entitled to Medicare Part A and enrolled under Part B, may elect to participate in a MSA plan.

   (b) Certain low-income Medicare beneficiaries are not eligible; namely, Qualified Medicare Beneficiaries, Qualified Disabled and Working Individuals, Specified Low-income Medicare Beneficiaries, or individuals otherwise entitled to Medicaid cost-sharing assistance under the Medicaid program.

   (c) To be eligible for a MSA, an individual must reside in the U.S. for at least one-hundred eighty-three (183) days during the year, and must not have permanent kidney failure or currently be receiving hospice care.

Chapter 6

Appendix C-5 Special Needs Plans
(continued)

3. **Bidding Methodology.**

SNPs have to prepare and submit bids like other MA plans.

4. **Payments to SNPs.**

SNPs are paid the same as other MA plans, based on the plan's enrollment. There are no special payment features specific to special needs plans. However, a **risk adjustment payment methodology** is being phased in for all MA plans. Under risk adjustment, payments are more accurate because they reflect the health status of an organization's enrollees. Therefore, to the extent that a SNP enrolls less healthy beneficiaries, it will receive higher payments to account for higher risk health status.

5. **Prescription Drugs.**

SNPs must provide prescription drug Part D coverage. Enrollees are not allowed to obtain other Part D drug coverage.

APPENDIX D
MEDICAL SAVINGS ACCOUNT (MSA) PLANS

1. **Background**

   <u>Private</u> MSAs, established by employers for some time, have enabled employees to obtain and pay for high-deductible catastrophic health insurance polices. The private MSA, still in effect, has stimulated development of two <u>Federal</u> demonstration projects. <u>The first of these projects was authorized in 1996 under the Health Insurance Portability and Accountability Act (HIPAA)</u>. It created a four- (4) year pilot MSA program which, effective January 1, 1997, allowed a maximum of 750,000 Medicare beneficiaries to be covered by a high-deductible catastrophic health insurance policy, and to receive certain favorable tax treatment. <u>The Balanced Budget Act of 1997 created a second Federal demonstration project</u> called Medical Savings Account (MSA) Plan. Enrollment was available to a maximum cap of 390,000 Medicare beneficiaries. **Under MMA, MA organizations are <u>now authorized</u> to offer MSA plans as a permanent option; <u>the enrollment cap was eliminated</u>**. MSA plans are considered "local" plans.

2. **Eligibility.**

   (a) Individuals, subject to the limitations mentioned in items (2)-(4) below, who are entitled to Medicare Part A and enrolled under Part B, may elect to participate in a MSA plan.

   (b) Certain low-income Medicare beneficiaries are not eligible; namely, Qualified Medicare Beneficiaries, Qualified Disabled and Working Individuals, Specified Low-income Medicare Beneficiaries, or individuals otherwise entitled to Medicaid cost-sharing assistance under the Medicaid program.

   (c) To be eligible for a MSA, an individual must reside in the U.S. for at least one-hundred eighty-three (183) days during the year, and must not have permanent kidney failure or currently be receiving hospice care.

Chapter 6   Appendix D - Medical Savings Account Plans (continued)

(d) In addition, certain classes of Medicare beneficiaries (though they have Medicare Part A and Medicare Part B) <u>are not eligible to choose a MSA plan, namely</u>:

- Beneficiaries who have coverage benefits that cover the high deductible of policies, including an employer's group plan that provides this coverage.

- Beneficiaries who are retired Federal government employees and part of the Federal Employee Health Benefits Program.

- Individuals who are retired Department of Defense or Department of Veterans Affairs employees

3. **Enrollment.**

Eligible individuals may select a MSA plan at either of the following times: (i) at the time they become entitled to benefits under Part A and enroll in Part B (the selection will be effective at such time), or (ii) in November of each year (the selection will be effective on January 1 of the following year). The first time an eligible individual enrolls, he/she has until December 15 of the same year to change his/her mind and choose another Medicare health plan. Otherwise, the enrolled individual must stay with the MSA plan for one full year.

4. **Medical Savings Account + High-deductible Health Policy.**

The MSA plan is basically divided into two (2) main operational parts: a MSA, and a high-deductible health policy (HDHP). Under the plan, <u>Medicare contributes the following</u> payments: (i) a <u>lump-sum contribution (annual deposit) to the MSA</u> (an account described in section (11) below), which the account holder may use only for payment of qualified medical expenses, <u>plus</u> (ii) <u>a monthly payment by Medicare to the insurance company of the company's premium</u>, for the HDHP that the account holder has chosen. The money expended by the Medicare program for the annual deposit, plus the HDHP's monthly premiums, equals the same capitation amount that the Medicare would have spent if the account holder joined another MA health plan option.

5. **Annual Deductible**.

The MSA pays for at least the items and services covered under Medicare Parts A and B, and such additional health services as the CMS may approve, **but only after the enrollee meets the amount of the annual deductible** of a required HDHP by first using the annual deposit or his/her own money.

For the year 2007, the annual deductible was limited to be not more than $9,500, nor less than $2,000. For subsequent contract years, the deductible may not exceed the maximum amount for the previous contract year, increased by the national per capita Medicare+Choice growth percentage as defined in Section 1853(C)(6) of the Social Security Act.

The MSA plan counts towards meeting the annual deductible all amounts that would have qualified for payment under Parts A and B by the enrollee as deductibles, or co-payments (but not supplemental benefits), as if the enrollee had elected to receive benefits through those Parts.

6. **Tax-exempt Trust or Custodial Account.**

The MSA is a tax-exempt trust or a custodial account created for the purpose of paying qualified medical expenses solely of the account holder. The account holder pays for the medical expenses, using the annual deposit in the MSA and his/her own money until the annual deductible is reached. After that, the HDHP will pay some or all of the enrollee's qualified medical expenses.

Qualified medical expenses are expenses defined as such under the Federal tax rules relating to itemized Federal tax deductions for medical care. The expenses cover a broader range than covered by Medicare (e.g., prescription drugs).

The trustees or custodians of an MSA may be a bank, insurance company or other financial institution satisfactory to the Secretary of HHS. They will provide a form of check or debit card to the account holder so that he/she can access the account; and they will report any deposits and withdrawals on the account to the IRS at the end of the year.

7. **Choice of Health Professionals – Network or Non-network MSA.**

An enrollee's choice of health professionals depends on whether a MSA plan is a provider network plan or a non-network plan described as follows:

- Non-network MSA Plan: With this plan the account holder has the free choice of doctors and other health professionals to whom payment is made for qualified medical services that they render.

- Network MSA Plan: This is a managed plan under which enrollees must receive services through a defined provider network consisting of providers with which the MA organization contracts to furnish healthcare services to Medicare enrollees under the MSA plan.

8. **Qualified Medical Expenses – Account Holders Only.**

The MSA may only pay for qualified medical expenses of the account holder -- not those of a spouse or dependents. Expenses may not include any insurance premiums, other than those for: long-term care insurance, continuation insurance (so-called COBRA coverage) and coverage while an individual is receiving unemployment insurance. Qualified medical expenses cover a range of services not covered by Medicare -- e.g. prescription drugs, dental claims (including false teeth) and vision care (including eye glasses).

To the extent payments are made by the MSA for non-qualified medical expenses, these payments are included in the taxable income of enrollee.

9. **Prohibition Against Commingling of MSA Funds.**

MSA assets may not be invested in life insurance contracts, nor commingled with other payments, except a common trust fund or common investment fund.

10. **Prescription Drugs.**

MSAs are not permitted to offer Part D drug coverage. MSA participants thus must separately enroll in a prescription drug plan.

11. Contributions by Medicare to the MSA.

The only contribution that may be made to an MSA is a specified contribution by the Secretary of HHS to the MSA.

The contribution begins, and is made in a lump sum, the month and year that an individual's election for the MSA plan is effective. The amount of the contribution for that month and all successive months in the year will be deposited in a single lump sum (**annual deposit**) during the first month. If an MSA is terminated before the end of the year, the proportionate share of the lump sum deposited by the Secretary of HHS must be refunded to Medicare.

If the amount of the required Medicare contribution to the plan (i.e., the capitation) is greater than the cost of the high-deductible health policy, the difference must be deposited by Medicare in the MSA.

12. Prohibited Sales of Medigap and Other Policies.

Insurers are prohibited from selling to an enrollee of a MSA plan a Medigap policy that duplicates benefits to which the beneficiary is eligible under Medicare.

Insurers are also prohibited from selling policies (other than those specified below) to persons covered under an MSA plan that would provide coverage for expenses that are otherwise required to be counted toward meeting the annual deductible amount of the HDHP. Thus, the account holder may not carry health insurance that covers the policy's deductible. This prohibition does not extend to HDHPs that provide coverage for any of the following: accidents; disability; dental care; vision care; long-term care; liabilities incurred under workers' compensation laws, tort liabilities, or liabilities relating to ownership or use of property; specified diseases or illnesses; and, a fixed amount per day of hospitalization.

13. Premiums.

Unlike all MA plans (other than PFFS plans), **MSA plans are without limit on premiums** that maybe charged enrollees for Medicare basic benefits (Parts A and B). **The plan is required to**

accept the Medicare capitation (i.e., the amount of required Medicare contribution) to the plan as payment in full for such basic benefits.

If the premium under the MSA plan is less than one-half of the required Medicare contribution to the plan, the Secretary of HHS must deposit an amount equal to the difference in the account holder's MSA.

14. **Charge Limits.**

(1) **When a provider does not have a contract with the plan.** A physician or other provider who does not have a contract establishing payment amounts for services furnished to an enrollee of a MSA organization is required to accept as payment in full for covered services amounts that physicians or other providers could collect if the individual were not enrolled in such organization (i.e., <u>**the amount that Original Medicare fee-for-services would have paid to an enrollee if enrolled in Original Medicare**</u>).

(2) **When a provider does have a contract with the plan.** A physician or other **provider of services** who has a contract with the plan establishing payment amounts **for services furnished to an enrollee of a MSA organization is required to accept as payment in full for covered services the amount set forth in the plan's fee schedule.**

15. **Tax Treatment of MSA.**

(a) **During Life of Account Holder**.

<u>The following are not included in the taxable income of the account holder:</u>

- Contributions by the Secretary of HHS to the MSA are not included in taxable income.

- Transfers of one Medicare MSA from one trustee to another trustee are not included in taxable income. When multiple Medicare MSAs may have been created by an account holder, he/she must designate only one as the MSA.

- Distributions from an MSA used to pay qualified medical expenses of the account holder are not included in taxable income and cannot be taken into account as itemized tax deductions for medical expenses.

- Income earned on assets in the MSA are not included in taxable income.

<u>The following are included in the taxable income</u> of the account holder:

- Payments for medical expenses of the account holder's spouse or dependents, or any person other than the account holder are included in taxable income of the account holder; they are not qualified medical expenses.

- Distributions made for other than qualified medical expenses are included in income. To the extent that they exceed a prescribed limit, such excess distributions are subject to a statutory penalty; the limit can be different each year. (For example, for the year 2006, the limit was equal to the account balance of the MSA on December 31st of the prior year, less sixty (60) percent of the annual deductible of the HDHP).

(b) **Upon death of the account holder**.

The tax treatment of the MSA depends on which of the three (3) following alternatives applies:

(i) <u>Surviving spouse is designated beneficiary</u>. The surviving spouse may continue the MSA, as if the spouse were the account holder.

- No new contributions may be made to the MSA.

- Earnings on the account balance are not included in taxable income.

Distributions for qualified medical expenses of the surviving spouse or spouse's dependents <u>are not</u> included in income. Distributions for the surviving spouse or his/her dependents, other than for qualified medical expenses, are included in the spouse's income. They are subject to a penalty tax, unless the distributions are made after the surviving spouse attains age 65, dies or becomes incapacitated.

(ii) A beneficiary other than surviving spouse is designated. The MSA ceases to be treated as an MSA. The value of the MSA is included in the gross taxable income of the beneficiary for the taxable year in which the death occurs.

(iii) No beneficiary is designated. The MSA ceases to be treated as an MSA. The value of the MSA on the account holder's death is included in the gross income of the account holder's final income tax return.

APPENDIX E
PRIVATE FEE-FOR-SERVICE (PFFS) PLAN

There are several types of Medicare Advantage plans that are alternatives to the Original Medicare fee-for-service plan. The MA Private Fee-for-Service (PFFS) plan is one of the alternative plans.

1. **Definition.**

    A PPFS plan is a plan that:

    - reimburses hospitals, physicians and other providers at a rate determined by the plan on a fee-for-service basis without placing the providers at financial risk.

    - does not vary its rates for such providers based on utilization of the PFFS plan by the providers.

    - does not restrict the selection of providers by enrollees to only those who provide the services and agree to accept the terms and conditions of payment established by the plan.

    - may provide supplemental benefits (i.e., benefits in addition to items and services available under Parts A and B) and coverage of additional services that the plan finds to be medically necessary.

    - <u>unlike all other plans, except MSAs</u>, may provide for payment by enrollees of an extra premium for Medicare basic benefits in addition to the regular Medicare premiums. Beneficiaries are liable for the full amount of any premium that the plan may charge.

2. **Premium.**

    <u>Unlike all MA plans (other than MSAs)</u>, PFFS plans are without limit on premiums that may be charged enrollees for Medicare basic benefits (Parts A and B). The plan is required to accept the Medicare **capitation** (i.e., the amount of required Medicare contribution) to the plan as payment in full for such basic benefits.

3. **Charge Limits.**

When a provider does not have a contract with the plan. A physician or other provider who does not have a contract establishing payment amounts for services furnished to an enrollee of PFFS organizations is required to accept as payment in full for covered services amounts that physicians or other providers could collect if the individual were not enrolled in such organization (i.e., the amount that original Medicare fee-for-services would have paid to an enrollee if enrolled in Original Medicare).

When a provider has a contract with the plan. A physician or other **provider** of services **that has a contract, or is deemed to have a contract**, with a PFFS plan **must accept as payment in full for services** that are furnished to enrollees an **amount not to exceed** (including deductibles, coinsurance, co-payments or balance billing) one-hundred fifteen **(115) percent of the payment fee schedule rate as determined by the plan.**

A health provider is treated (deemed) as having a contract with the plan (i) if the provider furnishes services that are covered by the plan and (ii) if before furnishing the services the provider has been informed of the individual's enrollment under the plan and has also been informed of the terms and conditions for those services under the plan or is given the opportunity to obtain information on those terms and conditions.

4. **Services to Enrollees.**

The plan is required to provide its enrollees through its physicians and other providers of **services not less than all those items and services, other than hospice care, available under Medicare Part A and Part B.**

5. **Access To Services – Primary Care Doctor - Specialist.**

The organization offering a **PFFS** plan <u>must</u> demonstrate to the CMS that it has a sufficient number and range of health care professionals and providers willing to provide services under the terms of the plan.

The plan **must** permit enrollees to obtain services from any entity authorized by Medicare to provide for Part A/B Services, and agree to provide services under the terms of the plan.

An enrollee is not required to choose a primary care doctor, or to obtain a reference to see a specialist.

6. **Quality Assurance.**

The plan is **not** required to meet prescribed quality assurance requirements.

7. **Explanation of Benefits.**

The plan **must** offer enrollees of the plan an appropriate explanation of benefits that includes a clear statement of the amount of an enrollee's liability, including balance billing, for services rendered.

8. **Notice to Enrollees by Hospitals.**

The organization **must** require hospitals to provide notice to enrollees prior to receipt of inpatient hospital services, or other services, when the amount of balance billing could be substantial. The notice must include a good faith estimate of the likely amount of such balance billing.

9. **Prescription Drugs.**

A PFFS **may** choose to offer Part D prescription drugs, and if it does, enrollees are prohibited from utilizing other Part D plans. However, if a PFFS does not offer prescription drug coverage, enrollees have the option of selecting their own Part D plan, or not.

CHAPTER 7

MEDICARE ADVANTAGE OUTPATIENT PRESCRIPTION DRUG PLANS (MA – PDP)

I. WHAT ARE MA PRESCRIPTION DRUG PLANS?

The Medicare Modernization Act (MMA), which was enacted into law December 8, 2003, established a new **Medicare Part D program** for voluntary outpatient prescription drug coverage ("**Part D Drug**") under the Medicare Advantage (MA) plan benefits described below. The Centers for Medicare and Medicaid Services (CMS) has overall responsibility for implementing the Medicare Part D prescription drug benefits and rules.

A. What Are Part D Drugs?

A **Part D drug** is one that is approved by the U.S. Food and Drug Administration, for which a prescription is required, and for which payment is required under Medicaid. Biological products, including insulin and insulin supplies (syringes, needles, alcohol swabs and gauge) and smoking cessation drugs are also covered under Part D. MMA excludes from coverage those categories of drugs for which Medicaid payment is optional, such as drugs for weight gain, barbiturates, benzodiazepines and over-the-counter medications. MMA also excludes from Part D coverage those drugs for which payment could be made under Medicare Part A or Part B. A Medicare Advantage Prescription Drug Plan (MA-PDP) is offered through a Medicare Advantage organization that offers comprehensive benefits, including Part D outpatient prescription drug coverage.

B. What Is Included in a MA-PDP Drug Formulary?

A plan's drug formulary must include at least one (but often two) drugs in each approved category and class. CMS has developed **appeals** procedures which ensure that enrollees quickly receive decisions regarding medically necessary medications. Pharmacies will distribute or post notices that instruct enrollees to contact their Medicare prescription drug plan if they need a certain drug and the pharmacist informs them that the drug is not included in the plan's formulary. The plans may change their formularies any time upon giving a sixty- (60) day notice to the enrollee, his/her prescribing physician, pharmacist and CMS, of formulary changes. The notice must explain how an enrollee may request an **exception**. If an enrollee requests an exception, the plan must make its decision as

Chapter 7   Medicare Advantage Prescription Drug Plan
                                                                        (continued)

expeditiously as the enrollee's health condition requires after it receives the request, but no later than twenty-four (24) hours for an expedited coverage determination or seventy-two (72) hours for a standard coverage determination.

C.   May Medigap Policies Include Drug Coverage?

No. Insurance companies are no longer able to sell existing Medigap policies that provide drug coverage to Medicare beneficiaries who are enrolled in or eligible for the new Medicare outpatient prescription drug coverage. They are, however, able to renew the Medigap drug policies issued prior to January 1, 2006 for beneficiaries who do not opt for the new Medicare prescription drug plan; drug coverage will be eliminated from these renewed policies, and premiums will be adjusted. Beneficiaries with the new Medicare drug coverage can purchase Medigap policies that do not cover drugs.

D.   Can Medicare Negotiate Drug Discounts?

No. The MMA prohibits the government from negotiating discounts on drug purchases or otherwise interfering in drug pricing decisions.

E.   Does Medicaid Cover Part D Drugs?

No. Medicaid may not provide Part D drug benefits to dual eligibles.

F.   How Much Cost-sharing Is There for Part D Drug Coverage?

MA plans may offer Part D beneficiaries **standard drug coverage** or **alternative prescription drug coverage** described below

1. <u>**Standard Drug Coverage.**</u> The MMA established the following standard drug cost-sharing that Medicare Advantage plans may offer.

   - A monthly **premium** (approximately $25 (2008) which varies depending on the plan chosen).

   - A yearly **deductible** of $275 (2008).

   - 25% of the yearly drug costs of $2,235 (2008) representing the costs between $275 to $2,510 (**initial coverage limit**), which amounts to $558.75. The plan pays the other seventy-five (75) percent (plan cost-share), which amounts to $1,676.25 (2008).

- One-hundred (100) percent of the next **additional out-of-pocket expenses** of $3,216.25 (2008) in drug costs (sometimes referred to as the "**doughnut hole**").

(b) **Coverage Gap (Doughnut Hole)**

Medicare Advantage drug plans may have a **coverage gap** which is sometimes called the "**doughnut hole**." A coverage gap means that a Part D eligible must spend a certain amount of money for the cost of covered drugs while he/she is in the "gap." This amount does not include the plan's monthly premium that must continue to be paid while in the coverage gap. The most the Part D eligible must pay out-of-pocket while in the coverage gap is $3,216.25.

Once the plan's out-of-pocket limit is reached, the individual will have **catastrophic coverage**. This means that the individual pays only a coinsurance or co-payment for a prescription (e.g., $2.25 for generic or $5.60 for brand-name drugs).

However, if the Part D beneficiary is entitled to **extra help** paying drug costs, he/she will not have a coverage gap.

(c) **Out-of-Pocket Threshold**

After having spent $4,050 (2008) out-of-pocket (**out-of-pocket threshold**), the beneficiary will pay $2.25 for a **generic** or **preferred brand-name drug** and $5.60 for other drugs, or five (5) percent **coinsurance**, which ever is greater; the plan pays the rest.

The deductible, initial coverage limit and annual out-of-pocket threshold are indexed for inflation each year.

For ready understanding, the $4,050 payments by the beneficiary for **2008** are set forth in the table below:

- **Annual Deductible**	$275.00
- 25% Co-pay of $2,235 (representing costs between the $275 deductible and $2,510 **initial coverage limit**)	$558.75
Subtotal (annual deductible + co-pay)	$833.75
- Additional out-of-pocket expenses (doughnut hole)	$3,216.25
Out-of-pocket threshold	$4,050.00

2. <u>**Alternative Prescription Drug Coverage**</u>. Part D drug plans are not required to offer the standard benefit, but can offer alternative prescription drug coverage. It must be "actuarially equivalent" to the standard benefit. In other words, the value of the benefit package must equal or be greater than the value of the standard benefit package. In an actuarially equivalent plan, the cost-sharing varies through the use of such mechanisms as tiered **co-payments**. However, a plan that offers an alternative benefit package cannot impose a higher annual deductible ($275 in 2008) or require a higher out-of-pocket threshold ($4,050 in 2008) than required by the standard benefit. Plans can offer **enhanced alternative coverage** that my include changes to the deductible and the initial coverage limit, though the deductible cannot be higher than the annual $275 (2008) deductible. **Enhanced alternative coverage** under Part D might include coverage of some drugs excluded under Part D, or in the coverage gap.

<u>Note</u>: In addition to the standard drug coverage plan, Part D eligibles are offered a wide variety of MA drug plans which must abide by the above requirements but may offer variations such as **gap coverage insurance** (i.e., **the doughnut hole gap**), no deductibles, higher or lower co-payments, etc.).

The cheapest plan is not necessarily the best. Among things to consider are whether a plan carries a deductible, what it charges for co-payments on individual drugs, whether it covers drugs in a doughnut hole, the cost of the premiums, and whether there are restrictions on some drugs.

G. Is a Subsidy Program Available?

The MMA provides for deductible, premium and cost-sharing subsidies (called **extra help**) for prescription drug coverage for certain individuals with low incomes and resources. The purpose of the subsidy program is to assist Medicare Part D beneficiaries with limited financial means to pay for Medicare prescription drug coverage (see section III below).

In order to receive **extra help** paying for prescription drug costs individuals must meet specific income and resource limits.

Resources include savings and stocks, but not an individual's home or car. If an individual qualifies, he/she will receive help paying for the Medicare drug plan's monthly premium, yearly deductible, and prescription co-payments. Subsidy-eligible individuals do not have a coverage gap.

An individual <u>automatically qualifies</u> for extra help if he/she has Medicare and:

- Has, or becomes eligible for Medicaid benefit (see section III.A(2) below)

- Gets help from his/her state Medicaid program paying Medicare premiums (i.e., the individual belongs to a Medicare Savings Program) (see section III.A(3) below); or

- Receives Supplemental Security Income (SSI) benefits without Medicaid (see section III.A(3) below).

If an individual lives in Alaska or Hawaii, or pays more than half of the living expenses of dependent family members, income limits are higher. Puerto Rico, the Virgin Islands, Guam, the Northern Mariana Islands, and American Samoa have their own rules for providing extra help to their residents.

H. Are Persons with End-stage Renal Disease Eligible for Part D Benefits?

No. Persons with ESRD are excluded from taking part in the Medicare Part D prescription drug program. An individual who develops ESRD while enrolled in an MA plan may continue in that plan, however.

II. HOW DOES ONE ENROLL IN A MEDICARE ADVANTAGE PRESCRIPTION DRUG PLAN?

A. Does Participation in a Medicare Advantage Plan Require Enrollment in its Prescription Drug Plan?

In order for Medicare beneficiaries to take part in the Medicare Part D prescription drug program, they <u>must enroll</u> in a prescription drug plan. These plans are offered by insurance companies and other private companies and cover both generic and brand-name drugs. Those firms serving the fee-for-service Medicare population (Original Medicare) are called **Prescription Drug Plans (PDP), also known as stand-alone plans,** and those serving Medicare Advantage (Medicare HMO), enrollees are called **Medicare Advantage Prescription Drug Plans (MA-PDP).** A beneficiary who becomes entitled to Part B is **not automatically enrolled** in Part D. Enrollment in Part D requires the beneficiary to take affirmative steps to enroll and get Part D coverage. The beneficiary must first choose a drug plan from the options available in his/her area. Then, the beneficiary must enroll through the plan that he/she chooses. If the beneficiary is eligible for the low-income subsidy, he/she must file a second affirmation.

<u>To obtain Medicare drug coverage from a Medicare Advantage plan, an individual must join a Medicare Advantage plan that includes drug coverage. A Part D-eligible individual who is enrolled in a MA-PDP, or a PFFS which has drug coverage, must obtain prescription drug coverage through that plan.</u>

<u>All Medicaid dual eligible individuals must be enrolled</u> in Medicare Part D in order to receive drug benefits. Enrollment in Medicare Part D is a condition of eligibility for Medicaid. An individual will lose all Medicaid benefits for failure to enroll or remain enrolled in a plan. New applicants who are Part D eligible do not need to be enrolled in a Medicare PDP in order to open a Medicaid case. Once they have an open case, the state will send their name to CMS for **automatic enrollment** in a plan.

Dual eligible individuals (see section E below) who reside in nursing homes are required to enroll in Medicare Part D.

An MA organization may not offer prescription drug coverage (other than that required under Parts A and B of Medicare) to enrollees of a <u>Medical Savings Account plan.</u>

Chapter 7

Enrollment - MA-PDP
(continued)

The MA-PDP will issue <u>a prescription drug</u> card to enrollees which they must use when purchasing prescription drugs. They must use pharmacies that are part of their plan's network.

<u>Note</u>: If a Part D-eligible individual has <u>prescription drug coverage from a former or current employer or union</u>, he/she should contact his/her benefits administrator before making any changes to his/her coverage. If he/she joins a Medicare Advantage plan, such individual and his/her family may lose their employer or union coverage.

B.   What Are the Enrollment Periods?

There are **three (3) coverage enrollment periods**: (i) <u>the initial enrollment period</u>; (ii) <u>the annual coordinated election period</u>; and (iii) <u>special enrollment period</u>.

1.   **Initial Enrollment Period.** The **initial enrollment period** for individuals who are <u>first</u> eligible to enroll in Part D corresponds to the initial enrollment period for Part B, i.e., the seven- (7) month period running from three (3) months before the month the individual first becomes eligible and ending three (3) months after the first month of eligibility.

Initial open enrollment in Part D runs from November 15 through December 31, when Original Medicare beneficiaries may switch from Original Medicare to a Medicare Advantage plan or enroll in a stand-alone plan if they have not previously done so. **Rephrased**: Beneficiaries may remain in Original Medicare and receive prescription drug coverage through **stand-alone prescription drug plans (drug-only plans)**, or join a **Medicare Advantage plan** that offers comprehensive benefits, including outpatient prescription drugs. Beneficiaries who become eligible for Medicare may enroll in a Part D plan when they become eligible for Part A <u>or</u> Part B benefits.

2.   **Annual Coordinated Enrollment Period.** The **annual coordinated enrollment period** corresponds to the annual coordinated enrollment period for Part C and runs from November 15 through December 31.

3.   <u>**Special Enrollment Periods.**</u>

Individuals may be eligible for a **special enrollment period**, if:

- they did not enroll in Part D during their initial enrollment because they had other prescription drug coverage deemed to be **creditable coverage,** and they lose the creditable coverage;

- they were given incorrect information concerning the status of their other prescription drug coverage as creditable coverage;

- they were given incorrect information about enrollment by a Federal employee;

- they have Medicare and full Medicaid coverage or a Medical Savings Account program;

- they move out of a plan's service area;

- their PDP's contract with Medicare is terminated;

- they enrolled in a MA-PDP during the first year of eligibility and want to return to traditional Medicare and a stand-alone PDP; or

- they move into or out of a nursing home.

4. **Effective Date of Enrollment.**

Part D coverage becomes effective:

- the same month that Part A and/or Part B coverage becomes effective for individuals who enroll before their month of entitlement to Part A or enrollment in Part B;

- the first day of the next calendar month after enrollment for individuals who enroll after the first month of entitlement for Part A or enrollment in Part B;

- the following January 1, for individuals who enroll during the annual coordinated enrollment period; and

Chapter 7

Enrollment - MA-PDP
(continued)

- at the time specified by CMS for individuals who enroll during a special enrollment period.

5. **Involuntary Disenrollment.**

An individual may be involuntarily disenrolled from a drug plan for reasons similar to the grounds for disenrollment from a Medicare Advantage plan. These include: no longer living in the plan's service area; loss of eligibility for Part D; death of the individual; termination of the PDP; failure to pay premiums on a timely basis; and, engaging in disruptive behavior that substantially impairs the ability of the plan to arrange for or provide services.

C. **When Can a Beneficiary Change Plans?**

1. **Changes During the Annual Coordinated Enrollment Period.**

All beneficiaries may switch plans <u>once</u> during the Annual Coordinated Enrollment Period, which runs from November 15 to December 31. Enrollment becomes effective on January 1 of the next year.

2. **Changes During Open Enrollment Periods.**

Individuals enrolled in a Medicare Advantage plan also may change plans <u>once</u> during the open enrollment period, which extends for the first three (3) months of each year. An enrollee in a MA-PDP may use the open enrollment period (January through March) to change to another MA-PDP or to disenroll from the MA-PDP and return to Traditional/Original Medicare and a PDP. Someone who enrolls in a MA plan that does not offer prescription drug coverage may not change to an MA-PDP or to Original Medicare and a stand-alone PDP during the open enrollment period. The beneficiary must wait to change plans until the next annual election period.

3. **Ability to Change Plans During Special Enrollment Periods.**

Beneficiaries are eligible to <u>change plans mid-year</u> if they qualify for a special enrollment period described above (see section B.3).

Chapter 7   Enrollment - MA-PDP
                                                                    (continued)

D.   What Happens If a Beneficiary Fails To Enroll on a Timely Basis?

A beneficiary who does not enroll in a Part D plan within sixty-three (63) days of his/her initial enrollment period, and who does not have other "creditable" prescription drug coverage, must pay a **late penalty** if he/she subsequently enrolls in a Part D plan. The penalty is assessed at one (1) percent of the national average premium for each month of delayed enrollment, for the remainder of the time in which the beneficiary is enrolled in a Part D plan. Thus, a beneficiary who first becomes eligible for Part D at age 65, but who delays enrolling until age 70 may be assessed a sixty (60) percent penalty on his/her premium (5 years x 12 months x 1%). Since the penalty is based on a percentage of the average premium each year, the dollar value of the penalty changes as the national average premium changes.

Late enrollment penalties will not be imposed if a beneficiary maintains **creditable coverage** (i.e., for example: MA-PDP or PD coverage, Veterans Administration coverage, Medigap coverage, and most employer (or union) sponsor retiree plans). Should a beneficiary's existing drug coverage end or change and thereby cease to be creditable, he/she has up to sixty-three (63) days to enroll in a Medicare drug plan.

E.   What Is the Enrollment Process for Individuals Who Are Full-Benefit Dual Eligible?

1.   A **full-benefit dual eligible individual** under Part D means an individual who is determined eligible by the state for: (i) medical assistance under Title XIX of the Social Security Act under any eligibility category covered under a state plan; or (ii) medical assistance under the Act authorized for the medical needy, or permitted by states that use more restrictive eligibility criteria than are used by the Supplemental Security Income (SSI) program. This definition is narrower than the definition of dual eligibles in other areas of the Original Medicare program in that it excludes Specified Low-income Medicare Beneficiaries (SLMB), low-income Qualified Individuals (QI), and Qualified Disabled and Working Individuals (QDWI). (These individuals under MMA, however, are deemed full-benefit dual eligibles.)

2.   Under the MMA there is a process of involving <u>automatic assignment</u> into drug plans for individuals who are full-benefit dual

eligibles, who are eligible for Medicare and Medicaid and who do not choose a PDP or MA-PDP during the initial enrollment period. **Full-benefit dual eligibles** at all times are automatically eligible for a special enrollment period.

3. Dual eligibles cannot receive Medicaid drug coverage unless they join a MA-PDP or a Medicare stand-alone drug plan to obtain drug coverage. CMS must automatically enroll full-benefit dual eligible individuals who fail to enroll in a Part D plan into a PDP that offers basic prescription drug coverage in the area where the individual resides and that has a monthly beneficiary premium that does not exceed the low-income premium subsidy amount.

Full-benefit dual eligible individuals who are enrolled in an MA private fee-for-service (PFFS) plan, cost-basis HMO, competitive medical plan that does not offer qualified prescription drug coverage, or an MSA plan and who fail to enroll in a Part D plan must be automatically enrolled by CMS into a PDP plan.

4. Nothing prevents a full-benefit dual eligible individual from: (i) affirmatively declining enrollment in Part D; or (ii) disenrolling from the Part D plan in which the individual is enrolled and electing to enroll in another Part D plan during the special enrollment period.

5. For individuals who are Medicaid-eligible and subsequently become newly eligible for Part D, enrollment is effective on the first day of the month the individual is eligible for Part D. For individuals who are eligible for Part D and subsequently become eligible for Medicaid, enrollment is effective upon being identified by CMS as a full-benefit dual eligible individual.

III. ARE SUBSIDIES AVAILABLE FOR LOW-INCOME INDIVIDUALS?

Under the Medicare Modernization Act, subsidies to meet all or some of the cost-sharing payments (deductibles and co-payments) are available for certain Medicare beneficiaries with incomes up to one-hundred fifty (150) percent of the Federal poverty level. These **subsidy-eligible individuals** are divided into the following three (3) categories according to income or Medicaid status: (i) a **full-subsidy-eligible individual;** (ii) individuals treated (**deemed**) as full-subsidy eligibles; and (iii) individuals who are **other low-income subsidy individuals (partial-subsidy individuals)**.

A. Who Are the Subsidy-eligible Individuals?

1. **A subsidy-eligible individual** is a Part D-eligible individual who: (i) is enrolled in or seeking to enroll in a Part D plan; (ii) has an income below one-hundred fifty (150) percent of the Federal poverty level; and (iii) has resources at or below the thresholds set forth below.

There are two groups of subsidy-eligible low-income individuals. The first group is composed of persons who either:

- are enrolled in a prescription drug plan or MA-PDP plan;
- have incomes below one-hundred thirty-five (135) percent of the Federal poverty level;
- have resources below $6,290 (2008) for an individual and $9,440 for a couple (increased in future years by the percentage increase in the consumer price index (CPI));

or

are full-benefit dual eligibles, regardless of whether they meet eligibility standards.

The second group of subsidy-eligible individuals is persons meeting the same requirements, except that the income level is above one-hundred thirty-five (135) percent but below one-hundred fifty (150) percent of the Federal poverty level and an alternative resources standard may be used. The alternative resource standard in 2008 is $10,490 for an individual and $20,970 for a couple (increased in future years by the percentage increase in the CPI).

2. **A full-subsidy eligible** individual has full Medicaid status (full-benefit dual eligible), income below one-hundred thirty-five (135) percent of the Federal poverty level, and resources less than $6,290 (single person) or less than $9,440 (married couple).

3. **Individuals treated (deemed) as full-subsidy eligible individuals** are those who are: (i) full-benefit dual eligible individuals; (ii) recipients of SSI benefits, without Medicaid; **or** (iii) individuals enrolled in one of the following **Medicare Savings Programs**: Qualified Medicare Beneficiary (QMB); Specified Low-income Medicare Beneficiary (SLMB); or Qualifying Individual (QI) under a state's plan. These programs were previously referred to as buy-in programs. Several years ago however, the CMS named them collectively Medicare Savings Programs.

4. **Other low-income subsidy individuals** (non-deemed, **partial-subsidy eligibles**) are those subsidy-eligible individuals who (i) have income above one-hundred thirty-five (135) but less than one-hundred fifty (150) percent of the Federal poverty level and (ii) have resources that do not exceed, $10,490 if single, or $20,970 (2008) if married.

B. How Much Are the Premium Subsidies?

1. A full-subsidy eligible individual (including deemed individuals) is entitled to one-hundred (100) percent of the premium subsidy amount.

2. Other low-income subsidy individuals (partial-subsidy eligible individuals) are entitled to a premium subsidy based on a sliding scale:

- A premium subsidy equal to seventy-five (75) percent of the premium subsidy for individuals with income greater than one-hundred thirty-five (135) but at or below one-hundred forty (140) percent of the Federal poverty level.

- A premium subsidy equal to fifty (50) percent of the premium subsidy standard for individuals with income greater than one-hundred forty (140) but at or below one-hundred forty-five (145) percent of the Federal poverty level.

- A premium subsidy equal to twenty-five (25) percent of the premium subsidy for individuals with income greater than one-hundred forty-five (145) percent below one-hundred fifty (150) percent of the Federal poverty level.

C. How Much Are the Subsidies for Drug Cost-sharing?

Subsidy-eligible individuals, according to their category, receive different levels of subsidies to cover cost-sharing (i.e., deductibles, co-payments). The subsidies are set forth below. Premiums subsidies described in point (2) above are repeated here and earmarked with an asterisk (*).

1. **Full-subsidy Eligible Individuals.**

    The cost-sharing benefits for full-subsidy eligible individuals (see section A.2 above) for a definition of this group) includes the following:

    - No premiums*;

    - No deductibles;

    - No doughnut hole (the amount of out-of-pocket drug costs that standard benefit beneficiaries are required to pay once their initial coverage limit of $2,510 (2008) is reached);

    - $1.05 co-payment for generic drugs, $3.10 for brand-name drugs up to the out-of-pocket threshold of $4,050;

    - No co-payments after reaching the out-of-pocket threshold;

    - No co-payment for Medicaid recipients residing in a medical facility. A medical facility is defined as a nursing home, psychiatric center, residential treatment center, developmental center, intermediate care facility. Individuals living in other group residences such as assisted living programs, group homes and adult homes are subject to co-payments.

2.   Deemed as Full-subsidy Eligible Individuals.

Certain individuals are treated (deemed) as full-subsidy eligible individuals regardless of their actual income and resources. (For the definition of these individuals, see A.3 above.) The cost-sharing benefits for these individuals include the following:

- No <u>premium</u> if enrolled in a plan with a monthly premium at or below the low-income premium subsidy amount (referred to as the "benchmark" plan)*;

- No deductibles;

- No doughnut hole;

- Co-payments of $2.25 for generic drugs and $5.60 for brand name drugs, up to the out-of-pocket threshold of $4,050; no co-payments thereafter.

3.   Partial-subsidy Eligible Individuals.

Individuals who are not dual eligibles and are not deemed full-subsidy individuals may apply for the subsidy benefit. The following partial subsidy beneficiaries may apply for the low-income subsidy through the Social Security Administration.

(i) Medicare beneficiaries, who are not eligible for Medicaid, with resources less than $10,490 (for a single person) or less than $20,970 (for a married couple) and <u>income below one-hundred thirty-five (135) percent of the Federal poverty level</u> will receive the following benefit:

- No deductible;

- No <u>premium</u>*;

- Co-payments of $2.25 for each generic drug and $5.60 for each brand-name drug, once the out-of-pocket threshold is reached ($4,050).

(ii) Beneficiaries with resources below $10,490 (for a single individual) or $20,970 (for a married couple), and <u>income between one-hundred thirty-five (135) percent and one-hundred fifty (150) percent</u> of the Federal poverty level will receive the following benefits:

- A sliding scale monthly <u>premium</u>* (see Chapter 5 section VI.B(3));

- A $56 deductible;

- Coinsurance of fifteen (15) percent after the deductible, up to the out-of-pocket threshold of $4,050; the government subsidy for cost-sharing counts toward the out-of-pocket limit; and

- Co-payments of $2.25 for each generic drug or $5.60 for each brand-name drug once the out-of-pocket threshold of $4,050 is reached.

CHAPTER 8

MEDICARE SUPPLEMENTAL INSURANCE (MEDIGAP)

Introduction

Medicare Supplemental Insurance is colloquially known as **Medigap** insurance. It is insurance commercially sold to Medicare-eligibles that is specifically tailored to provide them supplemental coverage. Depending on the policy, <u>Medigap policies pay some or all of Medicare deductibles and co-payments</u> and may also pay for some health services not covered by the hospital deductible; coinsurance for hospital expenses after a sixty- (60) day stay; costs for the first three (3) pints of blood; annual doctor bill deductible; and nursing home coinsurance after the Medicare benefit expires. <u>The policies require, as does Medicare, that the services provided be medically necessary</u>.

Until 1992, insurers designed their own Medigap policies. **In 1992, Congress mandated that insurers can only issue <u>ten</u> (10) standard policies known as plans A-J, and starting in 2006 <u>two</u> (2) additional policies were (K and L) added.** Although the benefits are standardized, the premiums for the plans vary from insurer to insurer and from state to state. Insurers can independently decide which of the <u>twelve</u> (12) plans they wish to offer. With the exception of Massachusetts, Minnesota, and Wisconsin which each developed their own standardized plans before 1992, Federal law requires insurers in all other states to sell Medigap policies that are one of the standard twelve (12) plans.

The Balanced Budget Act of 1997 added two (2) other options to the statutory ten (10) standard Medigap plans. Plans H and J may be issued with a **high-deductible insurance policy**. This policy requires the beneficiary of the policy to pay annual out-of-pocket expenses, other than premiums, in the amount of specified deductibles, and also requires the insurance company to pay one-hundred (100) percent of the out-of-pocket expenses of covered beneficiaries, once the deductible has been satisfied in a year. For 2008, Medigap high-deductible policies set the high-deductible amount at $1,900; in subsequent years, increases in the amount will be tied to the consumer price index (see section III below).

In addition to standard Medigap plans, **special Medigap policies known as Medicare Select** are approved for sale in all states. **Medicare Select** is a managed care Medigap policy sold by private insurance

Chapter 8   **Medigap (continued)**

companies or Health Maintenance Organizations (HMO). It began as a HCFA (now known as CMS) demonstration project authorized in fifteen (15) states and now is approved for sale throughout the country. Medicare Select policies are available to beneficiaries who agree to use providers who are participants or a preferred provider organization (PPO) of an HMO. If a participant uses a non-network provider, other than for emergency services, the Medicare Select plan is not obligated to reimburse the participant's incurred deductible or co-payment. The benefits covered under a Medicare Select policy are the same as those offered under one of the ten (10) original standardized Medigap plans depending on which plan is chosen to be offered for sale by the PPO or HMO and approved by the individual state. The advantage of Medicare Select policies to the enrollee is that premiums are likely to be lower than those charged for regular Medigap policies.

This chapter will offer a general overview of:

- Key characteristics of Medigap policies;
- Basic or core benefits of Plan A;
- The benefits of Medigap plans B through L; and
- Medicare Select policies.

Chapter 8 — Medigap

I. WHAT IS MEDIGAP INSURANCE?

Medigap policies cover a variety of services that must be medically necessary, just like Medicare, in order to be eligible for coverage. The Medigap policies are referred to by a letter, starting with Policy A and ending with Policy L. Policy A is the basic package, constituting the standard benefits. Plans B-J include all core or standard benefits plus various additional benefits. Plan J is the most comprehensive and the most costly. Plans K and L are the least comprehensive and the least expensive. The larger the number of services covered, the more costly the policy will be.

II. WHAT ARE THE KEY CHARACTERISTICS OF MEDIGAP POLICES?

- **Free Review Period**. Applicants interested in purchasing a Medigap policy are able to review a policy for thirty (30) days, starting from the date the applicant receives the policy. Any applicant who is dissatisfied with the policy or changes his or her mind within this review period can cancel the policy, and the company must fully refund the premium that had been paid. In effect, applicants can take a **free look** for thirty (30) days.

- **Pre-existing Conditions, Guaranteed Issue, Open Enrollment Period**. Under Federal rules, during the six (6) months (**open enrollment period**) after obtaining Medicare Part B medical coverage, an older person cannot be denied a Medigap policy for any medical reason. However, coverage for a **pre-existing condition** can be delayed for up to one-half year except for applicants who have creditable coverage. The term "**creditable coverage**" means coverage of an individual under one of the general medical health plans, such as a group health plan, Medicare Part A or Part B, or a state health benefit risk pool. In most states, except for certain individuals who are **guaranteed issue** of certain Medigap policies, Medigap coverage can be denied by insurers on medical grounds if the applicant misses the six- (6) month open enrollment window.

- **Premiums**. Insurance companies use one of three methods to fix Medigap policy premiums:
    1) The premium may be pegged to an applicant's age when he or she enrolled (**issue age**) so that a consumer always pays the premium required of a person of the same age when the policy was issued. Thus, if an individual buys a policy at age 65, he or she will always pay the rate the company charges people who are age 65, regardless of the policyholder's actual age;
    2) Premiums may increase as the beneficiary grows older (**attained age**); or
    3) All beneficiaries in a particular area are charged the same amount (**community rating**); the rate is based on the demographics and health experience of the group.
- **Portability**. In some states enrollees' movement from carrier to carrier or from one type of policy to another is restricted; this is particularly so in the case of people with pre-existing conditions.

Chapter 8   Medigap (continued)

III. WHAT ARE THE BENEFIT PACKAGES OF THE MEDIGAP PLANS?

Included in the standard benefits package are the following (see also summary chart in section XI below):

PLAN A – **Core or Basic Benefits**

- Medicare Part A **hospital coinsurance for days 61-90**;
- Medicare Part A **hospital coinsurance for days 91-150** which count toward the non-renewable lifetime hospital inpatient reserve days;
- All charges for a total of **365 additional lifetime days of inpatient hospital treatment**;
- Medicare Part A deductible of the **first three (3) pints of blood** yearly;
- Medicare Part B's twenty (20) percent **coinsurance of Medicare-approved charges, including physician** fees after the deductible of $135 (2008) has been met; and
- Medicare Part B's fifty (50) percent coinsurance of approved charges for **outpatient mental health services** after the deductible of $135 (2008) has been met.

The additional benefits of Plans B through J are listed below with an indication of the plans that incorporate them:

PLANS B through J – **Additional Benefits**

- Part A **inpatient hospital** deductible (Plans B through J)
- Part A daily **nursing home coinsurance** for days 21 through 100 of skilled care (Plans C through J)
- Part B **annual deductible of $135** (2008) (Plans C, F, and J)
- **Preventive health care**

  Up to $120 per year for **preventive health services** not covered by Medicare as long as they are ordered by a physician (Plans E and J)

- **Part B excess doctor charges**

| Chapter 8 | Medigap (continued) |

> One-hundred (100) percent of **excess doctor charges** up to one-hundred fifteen (115) percent of Medicare-approved amount (Plans F, I, and J)
>
> Eighty (80) percent of **excess doctor charges** up to one-hundred fifteen (115) percent of Medicare-approved amount (Plan G)
>
> - **At-home recovery**
>
>   Plans D, G, I and J pay up to $40 per visit for no more than seven (7) visits per week over a maximum of eight (8) weeks for personal care services at home such as bathing, eating and dressing. The maximum annual benefit is $1,600. Personal care services are covered only in conjunction with skilled home health care covered by Medicare following an illness, injury or surgery, and the personal care must be ordered by a physician and can be used for up to eight (8) weeks after the Medicare visits stop.
>
> - **Foreign travel emergency**
>
>   Eighty (80) percent of **medically necessary emergency care during the first two (2) months of each trip outside the USA**, with an annual $250 deductible and a lifetime maximum benefit of $50,000 (Plans C-J).

IV. WHAT ARE PLANS K AND L?

Effective January 1, 2006, two new Medigap plans were added – Plan K and Plan L.

Plan K offers fifty (50) percent of cost-sharing under Parts A and B, except that the Part B deductible is not covered. One-hundred (100) percent of cost-sharing for preventative benefits is covered in addition to the hospital coinsurance amount, and the 365 lifetime inpatient reserve days. The annual out-of-pocket amount under Parts A and B is limited to $4,440 in 2008, as adjusted by inflation annually thereafter.

Plan L covers seventy-five (75) percent of cost-sharing under Parts A and B, except for the Part B deductible. All hospital coinsurance and cost-sharing for preventative benefits are covered, in addition to the 365 lifetime

Chapter 8   **Medigap (continued)**

III. WHAT ARE THE BENEFIT PACKAGES OF THE MEDIGAP PLANS?

Included in the standard benefits package are the following (see also summary chart in section XI below):

PLAN A – **Core or Basic Benefits**

- Medicare Part A **hospital coinsurance for days 61-90**;

- Medicare Part A **hospital coinsurance for days 91-150** which count toward the non-renewable lifetime hospital inpatient reserve days;

- All charges for a total of **365 additional lifetime days of inpatient hospital treatment**;

- Medicare Part A deductible of the **first three (3) pints of blood** yearly;

- Medicare Part B's twenty (20) percent **coinsurance of Medicare-approved charges, including physician** fees after the deductible of $135 (2008) has been met; and

- Medicare Part B's fifty (50) percent coinsurance of approved charges for **outpatient mental health services** after the deductible of $135 (2008) has been met.

The additional benefits of Plans B through J are listed below with an indication of the plans that incorporate them:

PLANS B through J – **Additional Benefits**

- Part A **inpatient hospital** deductible (Plans B through J)

- Part A daily **nursing home coinsurance** for days 21 through 100 of skilled care (Plans C through J)

- Part B **annual deductible of $135** (2008) (Plans C, F, and J)

- **Preventive health care**

  Up to $120 per year for **preventive health services** not covered by Medicare as long as they are ordered by a physician (Plans E and J)

- **Part B excess doctor charges**

One-hundred (100) percent of **excess doctor charges** up to one-hundred fifteen (115) percent of Medicare-approved amount (Plans F, I, and J)

Eighty (80) percent of **excess doctor charges** up to one-hundred fifteen (115) percent of Medicare-approved amount (Plan G)

- **At-home recovery**

    Plans D, G, I and J pay up to $40 per visit for no more than seven (7) visits per week over a maximum of eight (8) weeks for personal care services at home such as bathing, eating and dressing. The maximum annual benefit is $1,600. Personal care services are covered only in conjunction with skilled home health care covered by Medicare following an illness, injury or surgery, and the personal care must be ordered by a physician and can be used for up to eight (8) weeks after the Medicare visits stop.

- **Foreign travel emergency**

    Eighty (80) percent of **medically necessary emergency care during the first two (2) months of each trip outside the USA**, with an annual $250 deductible and a lifetime maximum benefit of $50,000 (Plans C-J).

IV. WHAT ARE PLANS K AND L?

Effective January 1, 2006, two new Medigap plans were added – Plan K and Plan L.

Plan K offers fifty (50) percent of cost-sharing under Parts A and B, except that the Part B deductible is not covered. One-hundred (100) percent of cost-sharing for preventative benefits is covered in addition to the hospital coinsurance amount, and the 365 lifetime inpatient reserve days. The annual out-of-pocket amount under Parts A and B is limited to $4,440 in 2008, as adjusted by inflation annually thereafter.

Plan L covers seventy-five (75) percent of cost-sharing under Parts A and B, except for the Part B deductible. All hospital coinsurance and cost-sharing for preventative benefits are covered, in addition to the 365 lifetime inpatient reserve days. The annual out-of-pocket amount under Parts A and B is limited to $2,220 in 2008.

V. DO MEDIGAP POLICIES COVER PRESCRIPTION DRUGS?

No. Starting in January 1, 2006, insurance companies are not able to sell existing Medigap policies that provide drug coverage to Medicare beneficiaries who are enrolled in or are eligible for Medicare outpatient prescription drug coverage. They will, however, be able to renew the Medigap drug policies issued prior to January 1, 2006 for beneficiaries who do not enroll in a Medicare prescription drug plan. The Medigap drug plan policies of beneficiaries who enroll in a new Medicare prescription drug plan will be modified to eliminate drug coverage, and premiums will be adjusted. Beneficiaries with the new Medicare drug coverage can purchase Medigap policies that do not cover drugs.

VI. WHAT ARE MEDIGAP HIGH-DEDUCTIBLE POLICIES?

The Balanced Budget Act of 1997 allows Plans H and J, two of the twelve (12) standard Medigap plans, to offer an optional **high-deductible insurance** feature as part of the benefit package. Before the policy begins payment of benefits, a high-deductible insurance policy requires the beneficiary of the policy to pay annual out-of-pocket expenses, other than premiums, in the amount of a specified deductible, and requires the insurance company to pay one-hundred (100) percent of the beneficiary's covered out-of-pocket expenses once the deductible has been satisfied in a year.

Currently, Medigap high-deductible policies set the deductible amount of $1,900 (2008). In subsequent years, increases in the deductible amount are tied to the consumer price index.

VII. WHAT IS A MEDICARE SELECT POLICY?

Medicare Select is a managed care Medigap policy sold by private insurance companies or HMOs. Medicare Select policies are available to beneficiaries who agree to use providers who are participants of a preferred provider organization (PPO) or an HMO. The policies are substantially the same as standard Medigap insurance. If a participant uses a non-network provider, other than for emergency services, the Medicare Select plan is not obligated to reimburse the participant's incurred deductible or co-payment. The benefits covered under a Medicare Select policy are the same as those offered under one of the twelve (12) standardized Medigap plans depending on which plan is chosen to be offered for sale by the PPO or HMO and approved by the individual state. Reduced benefits are provided for items and services furnished by non-network providers. The premiums for Medicare Select policies are likely to be lower than those charged for standard Medigap policies because of these reduced benefits.

VIII. DO ANY MEDIGAP POLICIES COVER HOME CARE?

Some Medigap policies (Plans D, G, I and J) cover some limited personal care services that are not medically oriented and are not covered by Medicare. However, personal care is covered only in conjunction with Medicare-covered skilled home health care, following an illness, injury, or surgery. As is the case with Medicare home care, the personal care must be ordered by a physician and can be used for up to eight (8) weeks after the Medicare visits stop.

Plans D, G, I and J pay up to $40 per visit for no more than seven (7) visits per week for personal care services at home such as bathing, eating, and dressing. The maximum annual benefit is $1,600.

IX. IS THERE AN EXCLUSION (WAITING OR ELIMINATION) PERIOD DUE TO A PRE-EXISTING MEDICAL CONDITION?

Prior to enactment of the Balanced Budget Act of 1997 (Act), if a Medigap policy was purchased during the one-time six- (6) month **open enrollment** period permitted under the policy, an individual could not be turned down because of a pre-existing medical condition. However, the policy might impose a waiting (elimination) period (**exclusion period**), not exceeding six (6) months, before coverage for the pre-existing condition would take effect.

Under the Act, if an application for a Medigap policy is made **during the initial six- (6) month open enrollment period, an exclusion or waiting (elimination) period for a pre-existing condition may not be imposed under certain circumstances**. Commencing July 1, 1998, the exclusion may not be applied to any individual who, on the date of application for Medigap enrollment, has had at least six (6) months of **creditable coverage**. Persons having fewer than six (6) months, of such coverage are entitled to have the period of any pre-existing condition exclusion reduced by the aggregate period of creditable coverage they have accumulated.

Creditable coverage, with respect to an individual, means coverage of the individual under any one of several medical health plans, such as a group health plan, Medicare Part A or Part B, or a state health benefit risk pool.

X. **ARE INDIVIDUALS GUARANTEED ISSUE OF PLANS A, B, C AND F DESPITE A PRE-EXISTING MEDICAL CONDITION?**

Yes, subject to certain conditions explained below. If an individual seeks to purchase a Medigap policy after the six-month open enrollment period, the applicant generally can be turned down due to a pre-existing medical condition. However, the Balanced Budget Act of 1997 created certain exceptions. Since July 1, 1998, **certain individuals are guaranteed** issue of certain of the Medigap policies despite a pre-existing medical condition and even if purchased after the six-month open enrollment period.

Four of the twelve (12) standard Medigap policies – A, B, C and F – are designed by the Act to provide such guaranty. **It applies to individuals, specified below, "continuously" covered by a health policy.** They may avail themselves of such guaranty, provided they enroll in one of the four specified policies no later than sixty-three (63) days after termination of their prior coverage.

The following individuals are considered continuously covered:

- Individuals whose supplemental coverage under an employee welfare benefit plan terminates.

- Individuals enrolled in a Medicare Advantage plan who disenroll for permissible reasons (e.g., termination of the plan's certification or a move out of the plan area) other than during an annual election period.

- Individuals enrolled in risk or cost-basis HMOs or Medicare Select policies who disenroll for the permissible reasons explained above. With respect to Medicare Select policies, there must be no state law provision relating to continuation of coverage for this provision to apply.

- Individuals whose enrollment in a Medigap policy ceases because of the bankruptcy or insolvency of the insurer issuing the policy, or because of other involuntary termination of coverage for which there is no state law provision relating to continuation of coverage.

- Individuals previously enrolled under a Medigap policy who terminate such enrollment to participate, for the first time, in a Medicare Advantage plan, risk or cost-basis HMO, or Medicare Select policy, and who subsequently terminate their enrollment in such a plan during any permissible period within the first twelve (12) months of such enrollment.

- Individuals who enroll in a Medicare Advantage plan upon first reaching Medicare eligibility at age 65 but disenroll from the plan within twelve (12) months.

In addition to the above, individuals who re-enroll in a Medigap plan, after the one-time test of a Medicare Advantage plan, risk or cost-basis HMO, or Medigap Select policy, may re-enroll in the same Medigap policy, if still available from the same issuer, as they had before trying a Medicare Advantage plan.

All Medigap plans must be offered without the pre-existing condition exclusion to persons who enroll in a Medicare Advantage plan upon first reaching eligibility at age 65, and disenroll from the plan within twelve (12) months.

Chapter 8

Medigap (continued)

XI. SUMMARY OF MEDIGAP BENEFITS

Benefits	A	B	C	D	E	F*	G	H	I	J*	K**	L**
CORE Plan pays 20% coinsurance for doctor's bills, co-payment for hospital days 61-90 ($256/day, 2008), days 91-150 ($512/day, 2008) plus 365 lifetime hospital inpatient reserve days.	√	√	√	√	√	√	√	√	√	√	√	√
BLOOD (first 3 pints)	√	√	√	√	√	√	√	√	√	√	50%	75%
HOSPICE CARE coinsurance or co-payments											50%	75%
HOSPITAL DEDUCTIBLE Plan pays $1,024 (2008) for first day, not paid by Medicare.		√	√	√	√	√	√	√	√	√	50%	75%
DOCTOR'S BILL DEDUCTIBLE Plan pays the annual $135 (2008) not paid by Medicare.			√		√					√		
NURSING HOME COINSURANCE Plan pays $128/day (2008) for days 21-100.			√	√	√	√	√	√	√	√	50%	75%
DOCTOR'S CHARGES BEYOND MEDICARE LIMITS						√	80%		√	√		
MEDICAL TREATMENT OUTSIDE THE U.S. Patient pays $250 deductible and 20% coinsurance. Plan pays $50,000 lifetime maximum.			√	√	√	√	√	√	√	√		
AT-HOME RECOVERY FROM SURGERY OR ILLNESS Plan pays for up to eight weeks beyond Medicare-approved home care. Plan pays for seven visits a week by doctor or licensed nurse, with a maximum of $40 a visit or $1,600 a year.				√			√		√	√		

Chapter 8   **Medigap (continued)**

Benefits	A	B	C	D	E	F	G	H	I	J	K	L
PREVENTIVE HEALTH CARE Plan pays up to $120/year for health care screening and other preventive services not covered by Medicare.					√					√		

√ means that the Medigap policy covers 100% of the described benefit.

* Plans F and J also offer a high-deductible option whereby the beneficiary pays the first $1,900 (2008 deductible) in Medigap-covered costs.

** After the beneficiary meets the annual out-of-pocket limit ($4,440 for Plan K in 2008; $2,220 for Plan L in 2008) and the yearly Part B deductible ($135 in 2008), the plan pays one-hundred (100) percent of covered services for the remainder of the calendar year.

CHAPTER 9

PRIVATE LONG-TERM CARE INSURANCE

Introduction

As discussed in Chapter Three, Medicare's home health care benefit is limited to people who meet the strict medical criteria imposed by the law. Patients who do not fit the definition of homebound or who need non-medical home care will not qualify, even if they are otherwise entitled to Medicare.

Medicaid, described in Chapter Four, is a program that is means-tested and is not an option for all patients. Many patients will not qualify for Medicaid because their income and other financial resources render them ineligible for the program. Medicare Supplemental Insurance (Medigap) and private health insurance are not intended to cover chronic conditions or long-term care. **Thus, while patients may be homebound, they must rely on other sources to obtain home care.**

To help protect people against the high cost of long-term care either in a nursing home or at home, the insurance industry began to offer long-term care insurance policies in the 1980s.

In 1996 Congress enacted the Health Insurance Portability and Accountability Act. It further regulated the industry so that private long-term care insurance policies are treated as accident and health insurance contracts with several favorable tax consequences.

The home care services covered by long-term care policies may include skilled, intermediate, and custodial care. Some policies limit coverage to services provided by skilled providers such as registered nurses and therapists. Other policies also include personal care provided by home care aides.

<u>Long-term care insurance (LTCI) policies are usually indemnity insurance</u> that pay a daily cash amount to the policyholder, unlike service benefits paid directly to the care provider. Also, unlike other health insurance, most LTCI policies are individual policies. Employers play a limited but growing role in sponsoring group LTCI available to employees, their spouses, and sometimes parents and other family members. Employees usually pay the full premium for policies. Some associations also offer their members group LTCI. Group policies do not necessarily provide less expensive premiums or better benefits than individual policies.

Chapter 9   **Long-term Care Insurance**
                                                                                                                                                  (continued)

        The Health Insurance Portability and Accountability Act of 1996 mandated that LTCI policies must contain certain provisions in order for the policies to qualify for special tax benefits.

        This chapter will offer an overview of long-term care policies, including:

- Common characteristics of long-term care policies;
- Trigger events and other limitations;
- Benefits and coverage options; and
- Tax-qualified policies.

Chapter 9

Long-term Care Insurance
(continued)

I. WHAT IS LONG-TERM CARE INSURANCE?

There are two main types of individual long-term care policies: **classic** and **integrated** policies. Both types are presently available. Depending on individual circumstances, one or the other may be more suitable. Medical underwriting requirements for the two types of polices can vary. Potential buyers must therefore compare various policies before they make a selection.

II. WHAT IS A CLASSIC LONG-TERM CARE POLICY?

A classic long-term care policy is usually for nursing home care with a rider attached for home health care. Some classic policies mention alternative form of care as a coverage possibility. Usually, this means that the company may consider payment at its discretion for care in an assisted living facility, as long as it is cheaper than nursing home care.

III. WHAT IS AN INTEGRATED LONG-TERM CARE POLICY?

Under this type of policy, a beneficiary purchases a "pool of funds" for flexible use. Once the condition of the beneficiary meets the qualifying criteria for coverage, she may use this pool of funds as best suits her care needs, including care at home, in a nursing home, adult day care center, or assisted living facility.

IV. WHAT ARE SOME OF THE KEY CHARACTERISTICS OF LONG-TERM CARE INSURANCE?

Long-term care insurance is a complicated product requiring critical decisions on the part of the consumer. The following are some of its salient characteristics:

- Coverage may include a range of long-term care services, both skilled and personal (custodial) care, ranging from home care to assisted living to nursing home care.

- Long-term care policies generally exclude coverage for the following: alcohol and drug abuse; Medicare/Medicaid reimbursable expenses; services performed by family members; services outside the United States; and assistance with instrumental activities of daily living, such as preparing food, bill paying and transportation.

- To be qualified for tax benefits, policies cannot exclude coverage by type of illness, treatment, or medical condition, or accident.

| Chapter 9 | Long-term Care Insurance (continued) |

- The period of coverage which purchasers can select may be for one to two (2) years; three (3) years; four (4) to six (6) years; ten (10) years; or a lifetime. The longer the period of coverage the higher the premium.

- Virtually all policies currently issued are guaranteed renewable. This provision precludes an insurance company from canceling a policy so long as the insured pays the required premiums in a timely fashion.

- **The most crucial aspects of long-term care insurance policies are the so-called "triggers" (prerequisite events which trigger coverage).**

V. WHAT ARE TRIGGER EVENTS?

There are usually three (3) triggers that can operate separately or can be linked in different combinations. The triggers are:

- The medical necessity trigger requires that a physician must certify that admission to a nursing home or the need for home care is due to illness or injury, or is medically necessary. Policies with this trigger specifically state that the insured does not need prior institutionalization or skilled level of care before being eligible for coverage.

- The cognitive impairment trigger requires that substantial supervision from another person is needed to protect the patient's health and safety in the home.

- The limitations in the activities-of-daily-living trigger will determine how many activities of daily living must be impaired before coverage starts.

To be tax-qualified, policies must contain a trigger for five or six activities of daily living. To receive coverage, the insured must need "substantial assistance" from another individual to perform at least two such activities. A doctor must certify that the impairment will last at least ninety (90) days.

Depending on the policy, the three (3) triggers can operate separately or can be linked in different combinations. The best policies treat the triggers as single, independent events, each qualifying the beneficiary for coverage. When this is not the case, a policy with an activities-of-daily-living trigger paired with a cognitive impairment trigger, for example,

Chapter 9   **Long-term Care Insurance**
                                                                                          (continued)

usually will not cover Alzheimer's patients who are cognitively impaired but who are not necessarily limited in their activities of daily living.

<u>Policies vary in which ADLs are identified as trigger events</u>, how many ADLs must be impaired before coverage starts, and especially in the definitions of ADLs. One policy, for example, may define bathing, one of the common ADLs, to include sponge baths outside a bathtub, while another policy might define it to mean washing in a shower or bathtub. Differences in definitions can mean the difference between having coverage or not. <u>Activities of daily living</u> consist of activities usually performed for oneself in the course of a normal day and are usually considered to be: mobility (e.g., transfer from or to a bed or chair); dressing; bathing; self-feeding and toileting.

Policy differences in the definition of "assistance" with ADLs are also critical. Assistance may be defined as <u>total reliance</u> on another person or as <u>supervisory assistance</u>.

VI. WHAT IS THE COST OF LONG-TERM CARE INSURANCE?

The cost of LTCI premiums depends on several factors, including:

- The type of benefits selected (home care, alternative care, home modification);
- The daily benefit amount that is selected;
- The length of the benefit period that is selected; the length of the deductible or elimination period that is selected;
- The age at which a person buys a policy; and
- Any special coverage features such as inflation or non-forfeiture protection.

All companies offer a **level premium** which means that an individual policyholder will continue to pay the same premium charged at entry age (when the policyholder first purchased the policy). In other words, a person who was age 65 when he/she bought the policy will continue to pay the premium charged all 65-year-olds, regardless of the insured person's current age. Premiums cannot change unless a company receives approval from a state insurance department to increase the rate for an entire class of policyholders.

After an insured has received long-term care services for a designated period of time, most policies **waive** payment of premiums. Some policies count the elimination or waiting period when calculating the start of the waiver; others start counting after the elimination or waiting period. Most policies with this provision waive premiums after ninety (90) to one-hundred eighty (180) days. **Tax-qualified policies must have a waiver of premium provision.**

VII. IS THERE A PENALTY FOR NON-PAYMENT OF PREMIUMS?

Yes. If a policy holder does not pay the premiums regularly, the policy may lapse, and the insurance company may not reinstate the policyholder at the same rate. A policy may lapse when:

- The policyholder affirmatively decides to cancel it;
- Can no longer afford the premiums; or
- Simply forgets to pay the premiums for so long that the period of reinstatement expires.

In the event of an unintended lapse (for instance, when a policyholder suffers from a cognitive impairment or loss of function capacity and forgets to pay the premium), the policy can be reinstated if requested within five (5) months after termination, and if past premiums due are paid. Tax-qualified policies issued after January 1, 1997 cannot cancel a policy because a policyholder fails to pay a premium until thirty (30) days after written notification to the policyholder or a designated third party.

Some companies offer a **non-forfeiture benefit** for a higher premium, in case the insured lets a policy lapse. This provision provides that payments made on lapsed policies must be applied to purchase a fully paid reduced benefit or must be refunded in whole or in part. Without a non-forfeiture provision, premiums already paid on lapsed policies are lost. **To be tax-qualified, policies must offer an option to purchase non-forfeiture coverage.**

VIII. WHAT ARE THE BENEFITS OF LONG-TERM CARE INSURANCE?

Depending on the policy, long-term care insurance provides a predetermined amount of money per day, subject to an aggregate total, for services ranging from home care to nursing home care. Thus, policies provide a benefit limit based upon a dollar limitation, the number of days of covered care, or a number of visits by service providers.

Many long-term care insurance policies have a lower maximum benefit for home care than for nursing home care. For example, the selected home care benefit may be limited to fifty (50) percent of the maximum for a skilled nursing facility benefit. Or the duration of home care benefits may be limited to two years, whereas the maximum period of coverage for care as an inpatient in a skilled nursing facility may be four years. An optimum insurance policy provides at least the same level of reimbursement and duration of benefits for home care as for nursing home care.

Because LTCI benefits may be used at some future date when long-term care costs will likely be higher than when a policy is first purchased, many companies offer **inflation protection** (automatic percentage increases in the daily benefit amount) for higher premiums. There are three (3) ways of protecting against inflation:

- An automatic percentage increase in the daily benefit amount compounded annually. The higher the percentage of inflation rate selected by the policyholder, the higher the premium.

- A provision to have the daily benefit amount increase annually at a simple percentage rate.

- The option to purchase additional insurance based upon the consumer price index.

LTCI policies issued by the National Association of Insurance Commissioners provide for a five (5) percent compounded inflation protection.

IX. DO LONG-TERM CARE POLICIES INCLUDE A DEDUCTIBLE BEFORE PAYMENTS BEGIN?

Yes. Much like a deductible with other insurance policies, long-term care insurance policies impose an **elimination** or **waiting period** before paying benefits. Once an insured becomes eligible to receive benefits, as determined by the trigger event, he/she must wait a pre-selected period of time until the first benefit is paid. Consumers can elect an elimination period usually ranging between twenty (20) days to one year. The shorter the waiting period, the higher the premium.

X. CAN ONE BUY A LONG-TERM CARE POLICY WHEN THERE IS A PRE-EXISTING CONDITION?

That depends. Most older-long-term care insurance policies contain a provision disqualifying a prospective insured from obtaining coverage of a pre-existing conditions either permanently or for a specified length of time. To be tax-qualified, policies must define the term pre-existing to be the six- (6) month period prior to the effective date of coverage, so that a policy cannot deny coverage for a pre-existing condition after six (6) months following the effective date of coverage. Currently, major carriers issue polices that immediately cover a pre-existing condition so long as it is disclosed on the application form.

XI. CAN ONE UPGRADE A LONG-TERM CARE INSURANCE POLICY?

Yes, in some cases. Most long-term care insurance policies cannot be automatically upgraded. But policies vary. Some companies offer the right of an insured to upgrade without further underwriting medical examinations. When there is no right to upgrade, should a better policy later become available, the policyholder will have to apply anew for a policy, undergo a second underwriting medical examination, and pay a higher premium based upon his or her greater age or worsened condition in order to obtain the improved coverage.

XII. WHAT IS THE BENEFIT OF A NON-FORFEITURE CLAUSE?

Some companies offer, for a higher premium, a non-forfeiture benefit in case the insured lets a policy lapse. <u>This provision provides that payments made on lapsed policies must be applied to purchase a fully paid reduced benefit or must be refunded in whole or in part</u>. Without a non-forfeiture provision, premiums already paid on lapsed policies are lost. A policy lapses when the policyholder affirmatively decides to cancel it, can no longer afford the premiums, or simply forgets to pay the premiums for

Chapter 9	Long-term Care Insurance
	(continued)

so long that the period of reinstatement expires. <u>Tax-qualified policies must offer an option to purchase non-forfeiture coverage.</u>

XIII. CAN ONE REINSTATE A POLICY AFTER IT UNINTENTIONALLY LAPSES?

Yes, in certain instances. Tax-qualified policies cannot be cancelled because of a policyholder's failure to pay a premium until thirty (30) days after written notification to the policyholder or a designated third party. <u>In the event a policyholder suffers from a cognitive impairment or loss of functional capacity and the policy lapses, it can be reinstated if requested within five (5) months after termination and if past premiums due are paid.</u>

XIV. WHAT ARE THE REQUIREMENTS FOR A POLICY TO BE TAX-QUALIFIED?

A long-term care insurance policy must satisfy the following conditions to qualify for tax advantage as delineated under the Health Insurance Portability and Accountability Act of 1996:

- May not pay or reimburse Medicare-covered expenses except for **coinsurance or deductible amounts**;

- May not provide for cash surrender value or other money that can be paid, pledged or borrowed;

- Must contain a separate insurance coverage trigger for cognitively impaired individuals; and

- Must contain certain consumer protection provisions.

XV. WHAT CONDITIONS MUST BE MET TO OBTAIN TAX-QUALIFIED BENEFITS?

Under the Health Insurance Portability and Accountability Act of 1996 (Act), <u>LTCI policies are treated as **accident and health insurance contracts**</u> with several favorable tax consequences. To be eligible for these tax advantages, that is to be considered tax-qualified, LTCI policies and the patient must meet certain standards. In order to obtain tax-qualified long-term care benefits, a **<u>patient must</u>**:

Long-term Care at Home Consumer Guide

Chapter 9   **Long-term Care Insurance**
                                                                                                                  (continued)

- Be chronically ill, defined as:

    Unable to perform at least two (2) or five (5) or six (6) activities of daily living – eating, bathing, dressing, transferring from bed to a chair, toileting and continence – without substantial assistance from another individual (a physician must project that this disability will last at least ninety (90) days); or

    Requiring substantial supervision to protect him or her from threats to health and safety due to severe cognitive impairments.

- Need qualified long-term care services, defined as:

    Diagnostic, preventive, therapeutic, curing, treating, mitigating and rehabilitative services; and

    Maintenance or personal care services which are required by a chronically ill individual and that are provided according to a plan of care prescribed by a licensed health care provider. Maintenance or personal care services means any care or assistance with any disabilities that are a result of chronic illness, including severe cognitive impairment.

The policy:

- May not pay or reimburse expenses reimbursable by Medicare, except for **coinsurance or deductible amounts**.

- May not provide for a cash surrender value or other money that can be paid, pledged or borrowed.

- Must contain a separate insurance coverage trigger, independent of ADLs, <u>for cognitively impaired individuals</u>.

- Must contain certain consumer protection provisions set forth in the Long-term Care Insurance Model Act and Model Regulations developed by the National Association of Insurance Commissioners. These provisions relate to such policy features as an <u>inflation</u>

Chapter 9

Long-term Care Insurance (continued)

protection option, guaranteed renewability, and adult day care coverage.

If these conditions mentioned above are met, the qualified long-term care services are treated as a medical expense deduction for income tax purposes.

XVI. WHAT ARE THE TAX ADVANTAGES OF A TAX-QUALIFIED LTCI POLICY?

There are four (4) tax advantages associated with qualified LTCI policies.

1. Subject to limitations in amount, a taxpayer may treat LTCI premiums as un-reimbursed medical expenses and as such deduct them from taxable income to the extent such expenses exceed 7.5% of the taxpayer's adjusted gross income. The limits on deductions of annual premium dollars vary with the age of the insured. The 2008 limits, as set forth below, are indexed for inflation.

Age	Deduction Limits (2008)
40 and under	$ 310
41-50	580
51-60	1,150
61-70	3,080
over 70	3,850

2. Employers may deduct premiums they pay for policies offered through employee benefit programs.

3. Benefits received by taxpayers under an LTCI contract are excludable from gross income, subject to a cap of $270 per day (2008). The dollar cap is indexed for inflation according to the medical care cost component of the consumer price index. Per-diem policies must integrate long-term care riders to life insurance policies to meet the cap. If benefit payments exceed the dollar cap, then the excess payments are excludable only to the extent of the individual's un-reimbursed costs for qualified long-term care services.

4. Employer-provided long-term care benefits are tax-free to the employee. They are not excludable by an employee, however, if provided through a cafeteria plan of benefits. Expenses for long-term care services cannot be reimbursed under a flexible spending account.

XVII. WHAT ARE STATE PARTNERSHIP PROGRAMS FOR LTCI (ROBERT WOOD JOHNSON PROGRAMS)?

According to the so-called Robert Wood Johnson Long-term Care Program linking LTCI with Medicaid eligibility rules, if and when private insurance benefits are exhausted, the assets of policyholders are not counted in whole or in part (New York, California, Connecticut, Indiana and Iowa) in determining their Medicaid eligibility. However, all of their income will be counted.

Under some of the policies offered by the New York plan, a person who purchases a LTCI policy may establish his/her eligibility for Medicaid when the insurance benefits run out and thereby shelter an unlimited amount of assets from recovery by Medicaid. In the four (4) other states, a purchase of a LTCI policy will shelter assets on a dollar-for-dollar basis; the individual purchaser is able to retain an amount of assets free from Medicaid recovery equal to the amount of the LTCI purchased.

The Deficit Reduction Act of 2005 authorized all other states to adopt the foregoing program.

XVIII. CAN ONE OBTAIN MORE INFORMATION ABOUT LONG-TERM CARE INSURANCE?

Yes. Obtaining health insurance counseling before purchasing a long-term care insurance policy may be very helpful and cost-saving. Many communities offer health insurance counseling programs through their offices for the aging. In addition, private organizations, professional geriatric care managers and elder law attorneys are available in most communities to offer counseling and assistance.

CHAPTER 10

PRIVATE PAYMENT FOR HOME CARE

For home care here are two main approaches to privately paying to providers, namely (i) **direct contracting** with and payment to the care providers (for example, **direct hiring** of a nurse or attendant); and (ii) arranging care through and payment to a **home health agency**. Some people may obtain the services of a **geriatric care manager** to coordinate the foregoing services.

These matters are discussed in the following pages.

I. WHAT IS DIRECT CONTRACTING?

With the direct payment/contracting approach to home care, the person receiving the care, or a spouse, child, or other interested person on behalf of the care recipient, contracts directly with the individual provider(s) of care (e.g., nurse or health aide).

The person managing the care, whether the recipient, a family member, or a geriatric care manager, has direct control in the legal as well as the practical sense. This person may interview candidates for the job of nurse, housekeeper, or home attendant, and should verify the successful candidate's status as a citizen or legal resident alien. The person controlling the care may be delegated the responsibility for paying and remitting to the appropriate governmental agencies certain taxes: Federal and state unemployment taxes; worker's compensation or disability taxes; employer's and employee's share of FICA; and withholding taxes.

Among the advantages of direct hiring are:

— the ability to select the person best suited to care for the elderly person. Compatibility of personality may be as important as experience or technical skills; and,

— avoidance of the costs of a middleman such as a home health agency or employment agency.

— The possibility of having a privately hired home attendant certified for reimbursement by the Medicaid program once the care recipient becomes eligible for Medicaid.

The <u>disadvantages of direct contracting</u> (see section II below) may persuade individuals to obtain required services through home health agencies.

II. WHAT ARE THE ADVANTAGE OF USING A HOME HEALTH AGENCY?

The approach of <u>direct contracting</u>, including hiring, monitoring, and coordination of care services and related tasks, <u>entails the inconvenience of record keeping and taxpaying,</u> which can be significant. Many people feel unequal to these tasks and look to a **home health agency** (HHA) to perform these services.

The HHA, not the care recipient, is the employer and undertakes the responsibilities of employment. The agency will also arrange for replacement of workers who are unreliable or deemed unsatisfactory.

Patients requiring home care services may not qualify for Medicare coverage, but may choose (in order to have greater control of the selection process) to obtain nurses, home health aides, or other personnel from **licensed home care service agencies**. These agencies are private and licensed, but **not certified or covered by Medicare**. If the facility is licensed, it means that it has met certain minimum legal standards set by a local, state or government agency. If the facility fails to meet those standards, it could be fined, or in extreme cases, ordered to close. The fact that a facility is licensed will not guarantee that a person will receive high quality care. Because of tight budgets, enforcements of licensing standards are often sporadic.

A home health agency that is not a **Medicare-certified home health agency (CHHA)** may be less expensive than a HHA. On balance however, **it may be worthwhile to use the services of a CHHA because certification provides added reassurance due to the quality control effect of the Medicare conditions of participation and inspection**.

If a home care worker is hired privately through an agency, and the care recipient later qualifies for Medicare or Medicaid, (as the case may be) the home care worker's services can be covered by Medicare/Medicaid if the agency is certified for Medicare/Medicaid participation.

Chapter 10   Private Payment for Home Care
                                                              (continued)

III. HOW CAN THE SERVICES OF A GERIATRIC CARE MANAGER BE USEFUL?

Some patients or families, who are required or desire to resort to private payment for home care, whether they do so through direct contracting or a home health agency, may find it desirable to obtain the services of a **geriatric care services manager** (**care manager**) to assess the care required, and then obtain, screen, monitor and coordinate all of the care services. The care manager is in a position to work with care providers to help assure prompt and effective services to the patient (client), and relieve the caregiver (usually family members) of the formidable tasks of providing care.

The services of and the pricing by the **care manager** are described below:

- **Assessment**. Home care involves such decisions as: present and anticipated levels of dependency, living arrangements, care expectations, the family (or other caregiver) support system, safety of the patient in a given setting, and financial capabilities. Importantly, care management may call for the care manger to visit the patient's home to assess potentially critical current or future difficulties in terms of safety, space availability for health care equipment and homecare medical personnel, and suitability of bathroom facilities.

- **Development and Implementation of a Care Plan**. The care manager's services at the patient's or family's request <u>may</u> be an integral part of a comprehensive program. Once assessment of the patient's care situation has been completed, the care manager, with the assistance of registered nurses, <u>may</u> work with the patient's physician to design an individualized plan (program) of services to meet all of the clients' (the patient and their family) needs. <u>This individualized program</u> will include the appropriate combination of services such as professional in-home nursing care, either hourly or on a per-visit basis; personal care for bathing and grooming; complete live-in care; companion care; cooking, meal planning and marketing; laundry, housecleaning and errands; medical equipment and supplies; specialized care for Alzheimer's patients; escorts to medical appointments; modification of apartments or homes to accommodate the patient; and many other services.

- **Assistance with Placement**. If the patient cannot be reasonably accommodated at home, the <u>care manager may assist the family</u>

Chapter 10   **Private Payment for Home Care**
                                                                                                (continued)

<u>in determining the type of residential care facility</u> appropriate for and available to the patient and whether a skilled nursing facility, life care community or other type of assisted living facility is appropriate.

        The care manager, at the patient's or family's request, may review each potential facility with the client, arrange for in-person visitation, and accompany patients and family caregivers on these visits so that an independent evaluation and comparison of each facility may be made by the client. The care manager may assist in determining the quality of the facility, the services provided, any rating by an accreditation agency, the staff/resident ratio, its appropriateness for the patient (given social and temperamental considerations), the profit or non-profit status of the provider, and other areas of concern in selecting an appropriate assisted living facility or nursing home.

        After selection of a facility, the care manager may arrange for the preparation and the placement of the patient. The care manager may also by telephone calls and visits monitor the care provided to the patient. In order to alleviate any of the family's concerns regarding the facility, the care manager may prepare frequent reports. As the physical needs of the patient change, the care manager will continue to assess the patient's requirements in coordination with the patient's physician, and make further in-home or outside placements, when required.

        •   **Pricing**. The care manager may typically charge a flat sum of money for an initial consultation so as to become familiar with the patient's and family's crisis or other care needs; in turn, the family and patient familiarize themselves with the care manager's services and facilities. Thereafter, the care manager may charge an hourly fee for services, and/or possibly a flat charge for an assessment and preparation of a plan of care for overseeing the implementation of the plan.

CHAPTER 11

USING A HOME TO PAY FOR HOME CARE

Because Medicare and Medicaid will not cover all home care for all patients and since private long-term care insurance and Medigap insurance are costly and therefore not an option for everyone, patients may have to use their own financial assets to pay for home care.

This chapter discusses options available to homeowners to convert their home's equity into a source to funds to pay for home care.

I. WHAT ARE HOME EQUITY CONVERSION PLANS?

For many older patients and their families, the home is by far the greatest financial asset. As such, it is also an important resource for obtaining long-term care in the home or in a nursing home. Home equity conversion plans enable a homeowner to use the equity of his or her home to provide a stream of income over a period of years, while continuing to live in the home. There are two types of plans available in most states: **residential sale-leaseback** and **reverse mortgages**.

II. WHAT IS A RESIDENTIAL SALE-LEASEBACK?

Under a residential lease-back, the owner of the home sells his/her home at a discounted price to a third-party buyer/investor who then leases it back to the owner for life or until he/she moves. As part of the transaction, the buyer pays a portion of the purchase price in cash, and the balance by a note payable to the homeowner-seller, secured by a mortgage on the property for a stated term. The periodic payments, usually monthly, from the buyer are greater than the monthly rental from the homeowner-seller, and thus the difference represents a source of funds to the homeowner-seller to use as he/she wishes. At closing the buyer can take out an annuity which will pay to the seller for his/her life time, upon expiration of the mortgage terms, the same periodic payments as paid during the mortgage term.

III. WHAT IS A REVERSE MORTGAGE?

A reverse mortgage is a type of home equity loan obtained from a bank. The homeowner receives a sum of money from the lender (the bank), either in a single sum, in the form of a line of credit that can be drawn on at the homeowner's option, or in a series of regular payments. The plan usually takes one of two forms:

- A **short-term plan** under which a lending institution pays the owner of the home a monthly advance (loan) for a short period of time, and the owner of the home retains title to the home. The full amount of the loan is payable upon the maturity of the loan, at which time the home must be sold to repay the obligations. Thus, the homeowner, if he/she survives the loan period, must repay the principal and interest, or sell the house and move elsewhere.

- A **long-term loan** under which the lender receives not only interest on the amount loaned but also may share in a future appreciation of the property. (Some states will not allow shared appreciation.) The term of the loan is usually for a long-term (e.g., forty (40) years or greater) or for life.

Almost all reverse mortgages provide a guarantee of lifetime tenancy. Most reverse mortgages are non-recourse loans which means the lender can look only to the value of the house for repayment. **The homeowner retains title to the home** during the loan period. Upon the sale of the home by the owner, his/her move from the home, or his/her death (or earlier maturity of the loan), the loan and interest must be paid.

Some mortgages combine a reverse mortgage with an annuity, thereby guaranteeing individuals monthly income for their lifetime regardless of whether they continue to live in their homes or not. The monthly payments are considered annuity advances and thus partially taxable. For purposes of Medicaid eligibility, these payments may be counted as income.

With the passage of the **Home Equity Conversion Mortgage Insurance Demonstration Act of 1988** (HECM), lenders and homeowners, under a reverse mortgage placed under the HECM program, can be federally insured against default and eviction respectively.

IV. WHO CAN OBTAIN A REVERSE MORTGAGE?

To qualify for a reverse mortgage (either a HECM mortgage or non-Federal insured (i.e., proprietary) reverse mortgage), the homeowner usually must live in a single family home. There may also be certain minimum age requirements, varying by state. Typically, these age minimums are 60, 62, or 70 years of age.

As stated above, lenders and homeowners may be insured against default and eviction, respectively, under the HECM federally insured program. **To qualify under the HECM program**, the homeowner must be age 62 or over and live in a single family home. The maximum insurable amount ranges between $81,548 and $160,950. Loan applicants are required to receive counseling from an approved agency prior to obtaining the loan.

In addition to minimum age requirements, many states have other regulations concerning reverse mortgages. Prepayment penalties are barred. If only one spouse is a mortgagor, and the mortgagor spouse dies first, the surviving spouse is generally entitled to continue to reside in the home for life, and the mortgagee must wait for repayment.

V. WHAT IS THE EFFECT OF A REVERSE MORTGAGE ON MEDICAID ELIGIBILITY?

The states vary in determining whether a reverse mortgage will affect Medicaid eligibility.

- Several states (Colorado, Massachusetts, Minnesota, New York and Ohio) have laws providing that the **reverse mortgage** itself is **treated as a debt, not as an available resource.**

- In New York State, mortgage proceeds of a reverse mortgage are **neither income nor resources** for any purpose under any law relating to food stamps, public assistance, veteran assistance, Supplemental Security Income benefits and/or additional state payments, Medicaid assistance, any prescription drug plan or other payments.

VI. CAN LENDERS AND HOME OWNERS BE INSURED AGAINST DEFAULT AND EVICTION?

Yes. With the passage of the Home Equity Conversion Mortgage Insurance Demonstration Act of 1988 (HECM), **lenders and homeowners under a reverse mortgage, qualified under HECM to be HUD-insured, can be insured against default and eviction respectively.** To qualify, the homeowner must be age 62 or over and live in a single family home. The amount that may be borrowed is capped by the maximum Federal Home Administration mortgage limit for a particular area, which ranges between $81,548 and $160,950. The size of the actual reverse loan is calculated according to the borrower's age, interest rate, and the home's value. Older borrowers are allowed to borrow a larger percentage of their home's value. Loans which are made under this federally insured program require that loan applicants receive prior counseling from an approved agency.

VII. DO STATE LAWS REGULATE REVERSE MORTGAGES?

Yes. Many states have laws regulating reverse mortgages. In most cases, only persons over a certain age (typically 60, 62, or 70) can enter into reverse mortgages; prepayment penalties are barred. If only one spouse is a mortgagor, and the mortgagor-spouse dies first, the surviving spouse is generally entitled to reside in the home for life; the mortgagee must wait for repayment.

CHAPTER 12

ACCELERATED BENEFITS OF A LIFE INSURANCE POLICY TO PAY FOR HOME CARE

I. HOW CAN ONE USE A LIFE INSURANCE POLICY FOR HOME CARE?

Individuals who are insured under a **qualified long-term care insurance policy** and who are either **terminally ill** or **chronically ill** may gain access to a percentage of the value of death benefits (sometimes called **accelerated or living benefits**) covered by the insurance contract during life.

There are two methods by which the insured may accelerate death benefits of a life insurance contract.

- A **viatical settlement**: a sale by the insured to a viatical provider of a life insurance contract on the insured's life.

- An insurance company, pursuant to the provisions of a life insurance contract (or a rider to the contract), may directly pay to the insured during his/her life a percentage of the death benefits covered by the contract.

For purposes of obtaining these **accelerated benefits**, a terminally ill individual is someone who has been certified by a physician as having an illness or physical condition which can reasonably be expected to cause death in two (2) or three (3) months or less.

A **chronically ill individual** is someone unable to perform at least two (2) activities of daily living for at least ninety (90) days without substantial assistance or who requires substantial supervision to protect himself or herself from threats to health or safety due to severe cognitive impairment.

A qualified long-term care insurance contract is a guaranteed-renewable life insurance contract or a rider to a life insurance contract, under which the only insurance protection provided is coverage of **qualified long-term care services.** A qualified LTCI contract does not pay or reimburse expenses reimbursable by Medicare, except for **coinsurance** or **deductible** amounts. Nor may a qualified LTCI contract provide for a cash surrender

Chapter 12   **Use of Life Insurance Policy – Private Payment**

value or other money that can be paid, pledged or borrowed. Further, certain consumer protection provisions set forth in the Long-term Care Services Model Regulations and Model Act of the National Association of Insurance Commissioners must be part of the contract.

The Health Insurance Portability and Accountability Act of 1996 defines qualified long-term services as necessary diagnostic, preventive, therapeutic, curing, treating, mitigating and rehabilitative services and "maintenance or personal care services" which are required by a chronically-ill individual and provided pursuant to a plan of care prescribed by a licensed health care provider. The phrase "**maintenance or personal care services**" means any care the primary purpose of which is the provision of needed assistance with any of the disabilities as a result of which the individual is chronically ill, including severe cognitive impairment. **The cost of qualified long-term services can be counted as a medical expense deduction for income tax purposes.**

II. **ARE THERE TAX ADVANTAGES FOR USING LIFE INSURANCE DURING ONE'S LIFETIME?**

Yes. Under the Health Insurance Portability and Accountability Act of 1996, life insurance contracts are treated as accident or health insurance if the insured meets the terminally ill or chronically ill definitions outlined in section I above. If an insured who has a qualified long-term care life insurance contract is terminally ill or chronically ill, he/she may receive accelerated benefits tax free, **subject in the case of a chronically-ill person to a cap** and to certain conditions explained below (see sections III and IV). The amount of money received is excluded from the insured's gross income, as if it were paid by reason of the death of the insured.

III. **WHAT ARE THE CONDITIONS FOR A CHRONICALLY ILL INDIVIDUAL TO OBTAIN TAX ADVANTAGES FOR ACCELERATED BENEFITS?**

In order for a chronically ill individual to obtain the tax advantages for accelerated benefits, the benefits must:

- Be paid under the provisions of a qualified long-term insurance contract;

Chapter 12   **Use of Life Insurance Policy – Private Payment**
(continued)

- **Be for costs incurred by the insured for qualified long-term care services;** and
- Cover services that are not reimbursable by Medicare.

IV. WHAT ARE THE TAX ADVANTAGES OF ACCELERATED LIVING BENEFITS TO A CHRONICALLY ILL INDIVIDUAL?

In the sole case of a <u>chronically ill individual</u>, there is a dollar cap on the amount of accelerated benefits that can be excluded from income tax. The dollar amount is $270 per day (2008) or approximately $98,550 per year, indexed for inflation annually.

V. HOW DOES ONE OBTAIN ACCELERATED LIVING BENEFITS?

There are two methods by which the insured may obtain accelerated death benefits of a life insurance contract:

- <u>An insurance company</u>, under the provision of a life insurance contract, may <u>directly pay to the insured</u> during his/her life a percentage of the death benefits covered by the contract; or

- <u>A sale may be made by an insured to a viatical provider of the life insurance contract</u> on the insured's life, or the death benefits under the contract. The provider will pay the insured a negotiated percentage of the insured's death benefits.

VI. DO LIVING BENEFITS FROM A LIFE INSURANCE POLICY AFFECT MEDICAID ELIGIBILITY?

Yes. <u>Medicaid treats accelerated benefits as resources available to the applicant in determining Medicaid eligibility</u>. It is unclear whether the mere existence of a living benefits option makes an insurance policy an available resource for Medicaid eligibility purposes.

Chapter 12   **Use of Life Insurance Policy – Private Payment**
(continued)

VII. WHO IS A VIATICAL PROVIDER?

A viatical provider is a person regularly engaged in the trade or business of purchasing or taking assignment of the death benefit of a life insurance contract of an insured who is terminally or chronically ill. Such person must be licensed for such purposes in the state in which the insured resides. Or in the case of an insured who resides in a state which does not require the licensing of such person, he/she must meet the requirements of the Viatical Settlement Model Act and Long-term Care Insurance Model Act of the National Association of Insurance Commissioners.

VIII. WHERE DOES ONE OBTAIN INFORMATION ON THESE VARIOUS OPTIONS?

Patients and their families who need to obtain a home equity conversion or convert a life insurance policy in order to pay for needed home care should consult a lawyer who is familiar with these options and who is also knowledgeable about Medicare and Medicaid benefits. In each state there are elder law attorneys who specialize in lifetime planning and who are experts in tax law, public benefits, long-term care insurance, and trusts and estates. These experts are invaluable when a patient and the family need to plan for expensive long-term care.

CHAPTER 13

USE OF ADULT DAY CARE CENTERS FOR ELDERCARE OUTSIDE THE HOME

I. WHAT ARE ADULT DAY CARE CENTERS?

Adult day care centers provide frail elderly people living in the community a variety of services on a yearly basis (usually four (4) or five (5) days a week, approximately six (6) to eight (8) hours per day): recreation, social services, hot meals, frequent transportation and often medical, nursing and rehabilitative services. Programs which include medical services are state licensed. If programs provide no medical services, licensure depends on the particular state. Adult day centers sometimes provide transportation to their location.

There are basically **two types of programs** depending upon services rendered:

- Programs that emphasize social services, recreation, meals, and transportation. They <u>offer little, if any, medical services</u>.

- Programs, many affiliated with a healthcare institution <u>that provides medical care</u> and rehabilitation treatment, <u>in addition to meals, transportation, social and recreational activities</u>.

The National Adult Day Services Association (NADSA) has established **three levels of care,** or service, provided by adult day care programs: **core, enhanced, and intensive**. Participants in need of <u>core services</u> are those whose physical condition is stable, but who require some supervision, supportive services, minimal assistance with activities of daily living (ADLs), and socialization. Individuals needing <u>enhanced services</u> require moderate assistance with one (1) to three (3) ADLs, and possibly therapy services at a maintenance level. <u>Intensive services</u> provide maximum assistance, regular monitoring, or intervention by a nurse, and possibly therapy services at a rehabilitative or restorative level.

The New York State Office for the Aging defines adult day care as a community-based, nonresidential program providing four (4) core services for frail individuals: socialization, supervision, monitoring or personal care, and nutrition.

Chapter 13   Use of Adult Day Care Centers for Eldercare
                                                                           (continued)

II.   WHAT ARE THE FEES FOR SERVICES?

<u>The fee of adult day care centers varies from a flat fee to no fee, or a sliding fee depending upon the participant's income.</u> (In some adult day centers charges may be covered by Medicaid and in part by Medicare.) **Many long-term care insurance policies, where a fixed amount is paid for nursing home and home care, may include care in adult day centers as an additional benefit.**

Some corporations provide dependent care at an adult day care center covering parents of employees. This benefit is included as part of a cafeteria plan, and funded by salary reductions, thereby constituting a nontaxable benefit.

III. HOW DOES ATTENDANCE AT AN ADULT DAY CARE CENTER EFFECT ONE'S HOMEBOUND STATUS?

Regular absences to participate in therapeutic, psychosocial or medical treatment at a licensed or accredited adult day care program will not disqualify a beneficiary from being considered homebound for purposes of Medicare eligibility.

Home health agencies enrolling patients eligible for Medicare home health benefits are responsible for demonstrating that the adult day center is licensed or certified/accredited as part of determining whether a patient is homebound for purposes of Medicare eligibility.

CHAPTER 14

USE OF ANNUITIES TO PAY FOR ELDERCARE

Annuity contracts can be a source of private payment to an elderly person to defray or pay for long-term home care services <u>or</u> the costs of premiums of a long-term care insurance policy. They constitute a financial arrangement, such as an investment sold to an individual by an insurance company, under which, for a consideration, a continuing stream of payments is promised for the person's life, or for the joint lives of two (2) people or for a term of years to the purchaser or his/her assignee(s). The more common types of annuities are described below. An annuity contract may provide for payments to continue for a period certain (e.g. ten- (10) year certain) should the annuitant die before the expiration of the period. The annuity contract in some cases may provide for inflation factor.

I. WHAT ARE THE TYPES OF ANNUITIES?

<u>Deferred annuity</u>. A contract is entered into with the insurer whereby the insurer will commence payments at a specified date in the future, called the annuity start date. The purchaser of the annuity may either pay a single premium or an initial premium plus periodic later premium payments.

<u>Fixed annuity</u>. A contract is entered into with the insurer who agrees to pay a specified rate of return for a period of years.

<u>Immediate annuity</u>. A contract is entered into with an insurer whereby funds are transferred to the insurer. A single premium is paid, and an immediate stream of payments will begin.

<u>Joint survivor annuity</u>. A contract is entered into with the insurer who makes payments until the second of two annuitants, such as a husband and wife or parent and child, has died.

<u>Single life annuity</u>. A contract is entered into with the insurer who makes payments during the annuitant's life.

<u>Variable annuity</u>. A contract is entered into with the insurer with arrangements similar to those of a mutual fund. The annuitant is given a number of investment choices, and the annuitant's return will depend upon performance of the investments chosen.

II. WHAT IS THE TAX TREATMENT OF ANNUITIES?

The annuity recipient is not taxed on the portion of the annuity payout that represents his/her original investment. Taxes must be paid, however, upon any increased value of the annuity's accumulated balance resulting from interest, dividends or capital gains.

Usually until the original investment has been fully recovered, **each annuity payment will be multiplied by an exclusion ratio to determine the taxable amount**. The exclusion ratio is calculated by dividing the annuitant's investment in his/her contract by the expected return. The expected return in a life annuity is determined by multiplying the person's life expectancy figure, based upon Internal Revenue Code tables, by one year's annuity payment. In the case of a variable annuity, determination of the taxable amount of payouts is calculated in a somewhat different, more complicated manner.

CHAPTER 15

ALTERNATIVE HOUSING FACILITIES – PRIVATE PAYMENT

When persons reach a particular age or level of frailty, they often decide to move from their home to an alternative living situation, other than a nursing home for which such individuals must pay, that may better meet their changing physical and/or psychosocial needs. Alternative living facilities reflect the range of options that most often exist in the community; short of a skilled medical institution. Generally, they are residential in nature and incorporate a variety of psychological support and personal care services that may be required to permit an individual to remain living in that community, independent of a nursing home.

The facilities are best described by categorizing them into the levels of care provided by the facility where the resident lives. The facilities are described below.

I. WHAT INSTITUTIONAL, NON-MEDICAL FACILITIES ARE AVAILABLE FOR DEPENDENT RESIDENTS?

<u>Individuals who require some level of care, short of skilled nursing care, can reside in care homes in a non-medical, institutional setting</u>. Residents are supervised to varying degrees and are dependent to varying extents. These facilities range in size from a private home housing two or three seniors, to small facilities with approximately a dozen beds, to multi-unit complexes accommodating dozens of individuals. Licensure for these facilities varies by state. The facilities are known as:

Adult congregate living facility	Domiciliary care home
Adult foster home	Group home
Adult home	Home for the aging
Assisted living facility	Personal care home
Board-and-care home	Residential care home

<u>These facilities have no uniform definition around the country. Terms for them are fuzzy and lack a common meaning</u>. They may be called something different in a given state and also have a popular name that differs from a regulatory name. Thus, for example, a board-and-care facility is a lot

Chapter 15   **Alternative Housing Facilities (continued)**

like an assisted living facility, but the term sounds more déclassé and now seems to be used only in connection with a facility for low-income people.

An **assisted living** facility, commonly <u>less institutional than most of the facilities mentioned above</u>, provides a combination of housing and personalized health care in a professionally managed group-living environment designed to respond to the individual needs of persons who require assistance with activities of daily living.

The facility is specifically designed to promote maximum independence and dignity in the most residential and homelike setting possible. It may be all or part of a building that houses a few or several hundred persons, or a distinct part of a residential campus. It traditionally serves a resident who cannot or chooses not to live alone, but who does not require the twenty-four (24) hour skilled or custodial care of a nursing home.

Generally, residents of this type of housing pay privately in the form of rent, rent plus a fee or charge for services, and sometimes a deposit or entry fee. The price for services provided can vary specifically across the country. These services include: help hanging linens, and getting dressed, morning and bedtime care (hygiene, help in the washroom), registered nurse, dementia assistance, and access to concierge services in fancier facilities. Private long-term care insurance may be used for some of the provided services.

Licensure of this housing type varies by state, depending upon each state's own regulatory requirements.

II. WHAT NON-INSTITUTIONAL, NON-MEDICAL FACILITIES ARE AVAILABLE FOR SEMI-DEPENDENT RESIDENTS?

<u>For elderly persons who do not wish an institutional or medical setting</u> but require some minimal supportive services, there are several types of share housing facilities and arrangements. Examples include:

- Elderly owners of homes with housemate(s);
- Elderly persons who move in with relatives;
- Elderly persons who are matched up with younger persons and live in their homes;

| Chapter 15 | Alternative Housing Facilities (continued) |

- Foster homes for elderly semi-independent residents who move in with another non-related family that provides meals and other supportive services; and
- Accessory units.

III. WHAT NON-INSTITUTIONAL, NON-MEDICAL FACILITIES ARE AVAILABLE FOR INDEPENDENT RESIDENTS?

There are several housing options available to independent elderly persons who are basically well and capable of living independently, although they may have functional limitations. These individuals need only supportive services and amenities such as meals, health, transportation, and some social activities. The facilities suitable for independent seniors commonly consist of town houses, garden apartments or condominiums in which the resident generally has an equity interest, although sometimes these accommodations are on a rental basis. The cost of living in these facilities ranges from moderate to very expensive. These facilities are sometimes referred to as:

- Continuing care retirement community;
- Independent living retirement community;
- Life care community;
- Residential apartment; and
- Residential village.

The continuing care retirement community, and independent living retirement community are described in paragraphs 1 and 2 below.

1. **Continuing Care Retirement Community (CCRC).**

This type of housing alternative, sometimes called a life care community, generally requires that an individual be able to live independently upon becoming a resident in the community. As a resident begins to need more assistance, specific additional services are made available. Most CCRCs offer three (3) basic levels of housing on an as-needed basis: fully independent living, assisted living (personal care services) and skilled nursing care.

The basic idea of a CCRC is that once an individual becomes a resident, he/she never has to move again because any housing type and personal care services he/she will probably ever need are provided within the single campus setting. A CCRC guarantees housing and care across the continuum in that one community.

Generally, a CCRC will charge an entrance fee as well as a monthly payment for its residential, leisure and nursing services. In some cases, health care and personal care services can be paid for on an as-needed basis. The entrance fee, formerly nonrefundable, now is generally refundable on departure under a variety of specified conditions.

Basically, there are three types of CCRC contracts:

- ***Extensive contract*** covers shelter and residential services, amenities (e.g., swimming pool, possibly tennis courts and other types of recreation facilities) and unlimited long-term nursing care. The entrance fees and the monthly costs are usually higher than those under modified or fee-for-service contracts.

- ***Modified or fee-for-service contract*** provides shelter, residential services and amenities, plus a specified amount of nursing care, which the resident can obtain on an unlimited basis provided he/she pays for it at a daily or monthly nursing care rate.

- ***Fee-for-service continuing care contract*** covers shelter, meals, residential services and amenities, and in addition, emergency and short-term nursing care. Access to long-term nursing care is provided only upon a daily nursing care rate.

2. Independent Living Retirement Community.

Generally, this community is designed architecturally to be compatible with an older person's lifestyle, but offers no specific services beyond shelter, recreational activities and security. Most communities offer a variety of social activities and programs in an on-site clubhouse such as golf, tennis, swimming and other social amenities.

Structurally, an independent living retirement community can be built as single-family detached units, duplexes, mobile homes and other types of senior-oriented, low-density developments, or it can include apartment buildings and condominiums designed for older persons. It typically does not provide meals or other basic services due to the proximity to nearby community services.

Chapter 15 — Alternative Housing Facilities (continued)

Communities vary from independent ownership of units to monthly rentals depending on the individual community. While most are composed of private pay market-rate units, some rental apartment buildings may be subsidized.

Independent living retirement communities are also sometimes called retirement villages and communities, leisure or adult communities, residential apartments and residential villages.

IV. WHAT OTHER ALTERNATIVE HOUSING ARRANGEMENTS ARE AVAILABLE?

Several other types of housing alternatives merit mention. They are:

- **Accessory units**. Private housing arrangements in existing family homes, small cottages, or apartments that are in, attached to, or adjacent to living facilities. Examples of such units are ECHO units (see below), which are situated on the exterior of a single family residence, and accessory apartments which are created within the single family home.

- **Cluster care**. This is a cost-effective model of homemaker services for several senior residents living in a multi-unit housing complex. Traditionally, an individual contracts with an agency to provide the services of an aide for a minimum number of hours. With the cluster care model, one or more aides will service the needs of all home care recipients in one building, and thereby eliminate the need for an individual to pay for a minimum number of hours, and also allow an aide to revisit residents more than once a day if necessary.

- **Congregate housing**. One of the earliest defined types of housing with services. Congregate housing consists of a planned group environment offering the elderly who are functionally impaired or socially deprived, but not otherwise ill, the residential accommodations and support services they need to maintain or return to an independent lifestyle and prevent premature or unnecessary institutionalization as they grow older.

Congregate housing generally consists of individual apartments, in a managed multi-unit rental facility, with areas for group socializing and dining. Such housing caters to persons who are generally self-sufficient and mobile, who require no special care, but who choose to have certain services provided (e.g., meals, periodic housekeeping, transportation, social amenities and activities) that will encourage and promote independence.

Congregate housing facilities usually provide more extensive professional services than either board and care homes or shared housing arrangements. They are most often built with Federal, state and/or local government financing, and range in size from smaller projects containing twenty-five (25) to thirty (30) units to complexes with some three-hundred (300) apartments. Licensure for this housing type varies by state.

- **Elder cottage housing opportunity (ECHO) unit.** Sometimes called a "granny flat" or "in-law apartment," this unit is a small, manufactured home that can be installed in the back or side of a single-family residence and removed when it is no longer needed. It is designed specifically for older persons and persons with disabilities and is intended to enable them to live close to their family or younger friends, who will provide the support necessary for the older adult to live independently. The addition of an ECHO unit to an existing house or property is contingent upon local zoning regulations.

- **Naturally occurring retirement community (NORC).** An apartment building, complex or community, in which, due to the longevity of the residents and their aging in place, the majority of the residents are sixty (60) years of age or older. In such situations, an informal support system may develop where residents look out for one another. Recently, more formal comprehensive and accessible supportive services programs have become available to insure that residents do no "fall through the

Chapter 15

Alternative Housing Facilities
(continued)

cracks" of public benefits and other private service systems.

- **Shared housing**. This type of housing offers two (2) or more unrelated persons who are basically independent but who cannot or choose not to live alone the opportunity to share living quarters. Often, public or private community agencies own or operate houses or large apartments that house persons who have their own sleeping quarters, but share the rest of the rooms in the house or apartment.

   Private individuals may also make rooms in their own homes available to other persons in return for rent, services or a combination of both. A distinct advantage of this housing type is that it enables homeowners to remain in their neighborhoods and promotes community and neighborhood stability.

   While shared housing residents do not require residential or in-home health care, they do benefit by sharing household finances, cooking, shopping, housekeeping and other minimal support services which help them continue living independently.

   There are two distinct models of shared housing:

   — The match-up model pairs a homeowner or apartment dweller with a home seeker.

   — The group-shared residence, sometimes called a group home, houses three (3) or more persons living together as an unrelated family, sharing the responsibilities of making household decisions and pitching in on chores to the best of their abilities.

CHAPTER 16

FEDERAL HOUSING AND SUBSIDIES

The Housing and Development Act of 1959 as amended is the landmark legislation that established a Federal housing policy for senior citizens and created prototype programs for supportive services and/or Federal housing subsidies. <u>To qualify for most Federal housing and/or subsidy program persons must be sixty-two (62) years of age or older and have incomes that do not exceed eighty (80) percent of the median income for that geographic area.</u>

Several of the Federal programs are discussed below.

I. WHAT ARE THE MOST FREQUENTLY USED FEDERAL HOUSING SUBSIDY HOUSING PROGRAMS?

Several of the Federal programs under the Act are described below.

A. What Is the Section 8 Rental Subsidy Program (Voucher Program)?

This section has been the **most frequently used rental subsidy program** available and is widely used in public housing. It authorizes a variety of housing assistance programs. The one most applicable to the elderly is the Voucher Program (previously known as the Certificate Program).

The salient aspects of the subsidy program are set forth below.

1. **Administration of Voucher Program**. In the U.S. Department of Housing and Urban Development (HUD) **Housing Choice Voucher Program** (voucher program), HUD pays rental subsidies so that eligible families can afford decent, safe and sanitary housing. The program is generally administered by state or local governmental entities called **public housing agencies** (PHA). HUD provides housing assistance funds to the PHA. HUD also provides funds for PHA administration of the programs.

2. **Available Housing Types.** Several housing types are available under the Section 8 program, from single-family homes to high-rise apartment complexes. Vouchers can be used for a variety of housing,

including shared and manufactured housing, single-room occupancy units, group homes, and cooperative housing. Sometimes Section 8 housing units are available in congregate housing complexes for the elderly. Rental assistance is also available for assisted living provided the assisted living facility is the principal place of residence.

3. **PHA Contracts with Housing Owners.** Families select an available rent unit that meets program housing quality standards. If the PHA approves a family's unit, the PHA contracts with the owner to make rent subsidy payments on behalf of the family.

4. **Amount of Rent Subsidy.** In the voucher program, the rental subsidy is determined by a formula based on the local payment standard, which is a reflection of the cost to lease that particular unit in the housing market where it is located. If the rent is less than this standard, the family usually will pay thirty (30) percent of their adjusted monthly income for the rent. If the rent is more than the standard, then the family pays a greater share of the rent.

5. **Tenant-based Assistance.** As stated above, to receive tenant-based assistance, the family selects a suitable unit and an owner who is willing to participate in the program. After approving the tenancy, the PHA enters into a contract to make rental subsidy payments to the owner to subsidize occupancy by the family. The PHA contract with the owner only covers a single unit and a specific assisted family. If the family moves out of the leased unit, the contract with the owner terminates. The family may move to another unit with continued assistance so long as the family complies with program requirements.

6. **Eligibility.**
    (i) **General.** The applicant must be: a family, income-eligible and a citizen or a non-citizen who has eligible immigration status.

    (ii) **Income Requirement.** The applicant must meet certain income limitations. These generally require that the applicant's income not exceed eighty (80) percent of the median income in the area, adjusted for family size. The housing program does not have an asset or resource limit. If a tenant's total assets exceed $5,000, the amount

Chapter 16

Federal Housing and Subsidies
(continued)

included in his/her annual income is the greater of the actual income from his/her assets or a HUD-determined imputed income. Most types of income count in making this calculation, including Social Security and disability benefits, pensions, annuities, alimony, and regular contributions from others. Income does not include food stamps, reimbursements, specifically for medical expenses, one-time or infrequent income, and lump-sum acquisitions (e.g., inheritances, insurance payments, capital gains). There is a $400 standard deduction from annual income for an elderly family, as well as a medical expense deduction.

(iii) **Applicant Status.** An applicant must be:

- A family consisting of the applicant and one or more other family members;

- Elderly (i.e., age 62 or over);

- A disabled individual; or

- Two or more elderly, disabled or handicapped persons living together or one or more such persons living with another person who is needed to care for the dependent individual. A family that consists of one or more elderly or disabled persons may request that the PHA approve a live-in aide to reside in the unit and provide necessary supportive services for a family member who is a person with disabilities.

B. What Is the Section 202 Program of Supportive Housing for the Elderly?

This section provides one-hundred (100) percent of the **funds to community-based non-profit sponsors** to construct and operate rental apartment housing for "households" of low-income older persons. **Household** is defined as one or more people who are at least 62 years old or older at the time of occupancy. An earlier version of the Section 202 program included people with disabilities, but Congress created a new program, Section 811, for people with disabilities. Thus, elderly people with disabilities qualify for housing assistance under Section 202 or under Section 811. The program generally provides for a rental subsidy for eligible residents. The subsidy permits a below-the-market rate rent to be charged to eligible persons. The rents may not constitute more than thirty (30) percent of the tenant's income.

C. What Is the Congregate Housing Services Program?

This program provides funding to sponsors of senior housing for the inclusion of certain support services to be made available to residents of the housing project. Established in 1978 as a demonstration project, the program continues to be funded on a very limited basis.

TOPICAL INDEX
Home Care Basics

(References are to pages in Chapter 1)

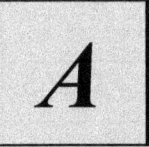

AVAILABLE TYPES OF CARE GIVERS	
Attendants	1, 7
Family members	1
Geriatric care managers	1
Home care workers	7
Home health aides	1, 7
Informal caregivers	1, 5
Non-medical persons	1
Private nurses	1, 6
AVAILABLE TYPES OF HOME CARE	
Activities of daily living	1
Custodial care	2, 4, 7
Dependent services in conjunction with skilled care	7
Home health care	1
Home maker/Housekeeping services	1, 7
Hospice care for the terminally ill	6
Instrumental activities of daily living	1
Medically oriented home care	4, 6

Topical Index (TI)
Home Care Basics
(continued)

Non-medical home care	1, 4, 6, 7
Nutrition services	6
Personal care services	1, 7
Physical and occupational therapy and speech-language pathology therapy	1, 6
Skilled nursing care	6, 41, 43, 265
Skilled services	1, 43-44

C

CERTIFIED HOME HEALTH AGENCIES (See also Sources of Obtaining Home Care)	8
COMMUNITY BASED AGENCIES (See also Sources of Obtaining Home Care)	13
COSTS OF HOME CARE	4, 5

D

DIRECT CONTRACTING	12

G

GERIATRIC CARE MANAGERS	1

I

INFORMATION AND REFERRALS	

Topical Index (TI)
Home Care Basics
(continued)

Adult day care centers	2, 15
Churches and synagogues	2, 15
Community-based organizations	13
Geriatric care managers	1, 15
Home health care agencies	2
Local office of Area Agency on Aging	15
National Association of Professional Geriatric Care Managers	15
National Elder Care Locator	15
Non-profit voluntary agencies	15
Public health and welfare departments	15
Senior centers	2, 14, 15

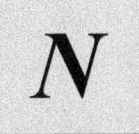

NUTRITION SERVICES	
Congregate meals	14
Food stamps	14
Home-delivered meals ("Meals on Wheels")	2, 14
Local offices of Area Agencies on Aging	14
Senior centers	14

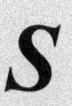

SOURCES FOR OBTAINING HOME CARE	
Advocacy assistance	13
Adult day care centers	2, 14, 25, 27

Area Agencies on Aging	2, 28
Churches, synagogues	2
Community-based organizations	13
Direct contracting	12
Home health care agencies	14, 18
Licensed home care agencies	22
Senior centers	2, 14

TOPICAL INDEX

Where to Obtain Home Care

(References are to pages in Chapter 2)

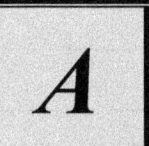

ADULT DAY CARE PROGRAMS	
Adult day care programs	25, 27
Home-bound individuals	27
Level of adult day care	26
Medical day care programs	25
Private pay	18, 22, 26
Social day care programs	25
AREA AGENCIES ON AGING	
Eligibility	28
In-home respite care	29
In-home services	28
Long-term care ombudsmen	29
Nutrition services	29
Senior centers	29

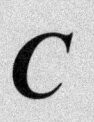

CERTIFIED HOME HEALTH CARE AGENCIES	
Home health aide services	18, 19

**Topical Index (TI)
Where to Obtain Home Care
(continued)**

Medical supplies and equipment	19
Nursing care	19
Nutritional counseling	18, 19
Personal care (home attendant services)	18
Screening of patients	20
Skilled nursing services	18, 19
Skilled physical, speech-language pathology and occupational therapy services	18, 19
Social work services	19
COMMUNITY-BASED AGENCIES	24

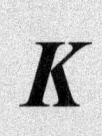

KEY SOURCES	
Adult day care programs	25-27
Area Agencies on Aging	28-29
Certified home health agencies	18-21
Community-based agencies	24
Licensed home care agencies	18, 22-23

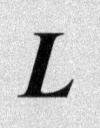

LICENSED HOME CARE AGENCIES (See also Certified home health care agencies)	18, 22-23

Long-term Care at Home Consumer Guide   © 2009 Walter Feldesman

TOPICAL INDEX

Medicare
(References are to pages in Chapter 3)

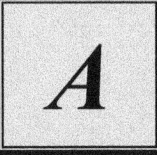

ADMINISTRATION OF MEDICARE	
Carriers, administrative duties performed by	31
Centers of Medicare and Medicaid Services (CMS), administrative duties performed by	31
Department of Health and Human Services (HHS), administrative duties performed by	31
Fiscal intermediaries, administrative duties performed by	31
Quality Improvement Organizations (QIO), administrative duties performed by	32
Qualified independent contractors (QIC), administrative duties performed by	32
Peer review organization	32
AMBULANCE TRANSPORTATION	
CAH hospital, coverage of ambulance transportation to	87
Medical necessity, physician's certification requirements	87
Nearest hospital/SNF rule	87
Part A coverage of ambulance transportation	87
Part B coverage of ambulance transportation	87
Renal dialysis treatment center, coverage of ambulance transportation to	87
SNF, coverage of ambulance transportation to	87

Topical Index (TI)
Medicare
(continued)

APPEALS OF PART A AND PART B CLAIMS	54-59
AUTOMATIC ENROLLMENT PART A (see also Eligibility and Enrollment, this index)	37
AUTOMATIC ENROLLMENT PART B (see also Eligibility and Enrollment, this index)	37

B

BILLING AND PAYMENT FOR PART B SERVICES AND SUPPLIES	
Approved (allowed) charges	72
Balance billing, limitations on	73
Institutional providers, payment procedures pertaining to	73
Part B billing procedures	72
Part B payment of bills	73
Processing claims where no assignment is made	72-73
Provider, acceptance of assignment by	72

C

CERTIFIED HOME HEALTH AGENCIES	44
CONSOLIDATED OMNIBUS BUDGET RECONCILIATION ACT (COBRA) OF 1985	64
Age 65 and older, employee's right to compel Part B enrollment	64
Employer medical insurance, continuation for 18 months after termination	64
Optional cancellation of coverage by employer	64

Topical Index (TI)
Medicare
(continued)

Termination of COBRA coverage upon Medicare enrollment	64
COORDINATION OF COVERAGE – EMPLOYER PLANS	93

D

DEDUCTIBLES/COINSURANCE PAYMENTS	
Amount of payments	71
Coinsurance (co-payment), Part B	71
DEMAND BILL	
Advance beneficiary notice	54-55
Fiscal intermediary, submission of demand bill to	55
Home health agency, submission of demand bill in non-coverage dispute	55
Payment for services pending review of demand bill	53
DURABLE MEDICAL EQUIPMENT (DME)	
Overview	47, 83-86
Capped rental items, purchase option pertaining to	85
Certificate of medical necessity, required signing by treating physician	84
Defined	83
Durability requirement for DME	83
Home oxygen services, Medicare coverage of	85
Items of medical equipment covered under Medicare	83
Maintenance of DME, Medicare payment for	84
Medical equipment, exclusion from Medicare coverage	83
Necessary and reasonable requirements	84

Part B coverage of DME	84
Physician's prescription for DME, necessity for	84
Prosthetic devices, defined	85-86
Repairs of DME, Medicare coverage of costs of repairs	84
Supplies and accessories, Medicare reimbursement for	85
Use in home, necessity for	83-84

ELIGIBILITY AND ENROLLMENT	
Age as basis for hospital insurance eligibility	37
Aliens, restrictions on Medicare eligibility	38
Amytrophic Lateral Sclerosis (ALS) ("Lou Gehrig's Disease"), eligibility based on	35
Application for enrollment, necessity for	37-38
Automatic enrollment as basis for eligibility (Original Medicare)	37
Dialysis/kidney transplant patients, eligibility	34
Disabled Social Security/Railroad Retirement beneficiary, eligibility based on	34
Federal employment, eligibility based on	35
General (annual) enrollment period, time period within to file	39
Initial enrollment period (Original Medicare)	38-39
Late filing for initial enrollment, penalty/surcharge imposed for (Original Medicare)	40
Period(s) of enrollment, necessity to file within (Original Medicare)	38-39
Qualified Medicare beneficiaries	36
Qualified disabled and working individuals	36

Topical Index (TI)
Medicare
(continued)

Qualifying individuals	36
Retirement of employees, continue private insurance	36
Social Security/Railroad Retirement benefits, receipt as basis for eligibility	34
Special enrollment period (Original Medicare)	39
Specified Low-income Medicare beneficiaries	36
Waiting period, 3-month waiting period requirement in dialysis cases	34

H

HEALTH CARE INSURANCE CARD	
Automatic mailing of card	32
Damaged card, securing replacement for	33
Entitlement, persons entitled to card	32
Lost card, securing replacement	33
HOME HEALTH CARE	
Overview	41
Absence from home as non-qualifying event	42
Types of home health care services provided under Medicare program	43-48
Certified home health agency, defined	44
Confinement to the home, defined	42
Dependent services, list of covered services under Medicare	44-48
Durable medical equipment, coverage under Medicare	47
Eligibility for home health services, qualifying requirements	41
Exclusions	49

Topical Index (TI)
Medicare
(continued)

Homebound eligibility requirement	42
Home care and home health care, distinguished	6
Home health services, defined	45
Home health aide services, coverage under Medicare	45
Home health agency (Certified home health agency)	44
Intermittent, defined	43
Intermittent skilled nursing care coverage	41
Intern/resident services, coverage under Medicare	48
Medical social services, generally	46
Medical supplies, coverage under Medicare	47-48
Medicare exclusions, list of exclusions	49
Occupational therapy, coverage in a home care setting	77
Part-time or intermittent	43-44
Payment by Part B	77
Physical therapy, speech-language pathology services, occupational therapy coverage in home care setting	77
Physician's direction, requirement pertaining to	77
Plan of care	42
Qualifying skilled services, coverage under Medicare	41, 43
Skilled nursing care, defined	43
Speech-language pathology services, coverage in home care setting	77
HOSPICE CARE	
Overview	51
Election of hospice care instead of standard Medicare benefits	51
Medicare-certified hospice program, necessity for	51
Physician certification requirement	51
Services and items covered under hospice program	52-53

Topical Index (TI)
Medicare
(continued)

K

KIDNEYS	67

L

LICENSED HOME CARE AGENCIES	
Nature of care furnished by home care service agencies	19
Non-Medicare certified agencies, obtaining home care from	22
Obtaining home care services from home care agencies	18
LOW-INCOME INDIVIDUALS	
Deductibles/coinsurance/co-payments/premiums (Medicare) payment by Medicaid	109
Dual eligibles (Original Medicare)	74
Income/resource guidelines for QMB beneficiaries (Original Medicare)	109
Low-income qualifying individual (QI-1), income/resource limits pertaining to	75
Qualified disabled/working individual income/resource limiting premium payments	75
Qualified Medicare beneficiary (QMB), buy-in to Medicare by Medicaid	74
Specified low-income Medicare beneficiary (SLMB), income/resource limits	75

M

MEDICARE AS SECONDARY PAYER	

Overview	60
Federal government, lawsuit by to recover conditional payments	60
Incorrect Medicare payments, three- (3) year recovery period	60
Primary payer, initial duty to make payment	60
Recovery of Medicare payments from primary payer	60
MEDICARE PRIVATE CONTRACTS (OPTING OUT OF MEDICARE)	
Overview	91
Private contracts, parties authorized to enter into	91
Private contract, prohibition against receiving Medicare payment	91
MEDICARE SUMMARY NOTICE (MSN)	
Appeal procedures contained in MSN	54
Contents of notice	54
MENTAL HEALTH SERVICES	82

O

OUTPATIENT SKILLED THERAPY	77-79

P

PART B SUPPLEMENTAL INSURANCE COVERAGE OF SERVICES	
Ambulance service	66
Blood clotting factors	66

**Topical Index (TI)
Medicare
(continued)**

Bone mass measurement	68
Chiropractor	70
Diabetes	67, 88-89
Diagnosis and treatment of eye and ear ailments	65
Durable medical equipment	66
Eyeglasses following cataract surgery	68
Exclusions	69
Flu shot	67, 70
Hepatitis B vaccine	68, 70
Immunopressive drugs	66
Injectible drugs for treatment of bone fracture	68
Intravenous immune gobulin	68
Kidney dialysis equipment	67
Mental health/psychiatrist care	66, 68-69, 81
Outpatient department hospital services	66, 81
Outpatient physical and occupational therapy and speech-language pathology services	66, 77-80
Outpatient rehabilitation services	66, 77-80
Plastic surgery to repair accident injury, impaired limb or malformed part of body	65
Pneumonia shot	70
Podiatrist	65
Radiation therapy	66
Radiological or pathological services	65
Reasonable and necessary requirements	42, 70-71, 78
Screening tests for preventive of disease	68
Transplants	67

Q

QUALIFIED DISABLED AND WORKING INDIVIDUALS	
Poverty level needed to qualify	75
Premium payment through Medicaid/Medicare	75
Qualifying individuals	36, 75
QUALIFIED MEDICARE BENEFICIARY	36, 74

R

Rehabilitation	66, 77-80

S

SERVICE ENTITLEMENT BASED ON MEDICARE CARD	
Automatic mailing of Medicare card	32
Color of Medicare card	32
Part A and Part B benefits based on Medicare card	32
Replacement of damaged/lost Medicare card	33
SERVICES COVERED (see also Part B supplemental insurance coverage of services)	65

TOPICAL INDEX

Medicaid

(References are to pages in Chapter 4)

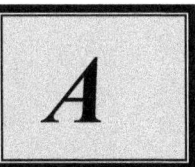

APPEALS PROCESS	
De novo hearing	127
fair hearing	127
time limitations	127
written notice, right to	127
ALIENS, STATUS OF	96, 98

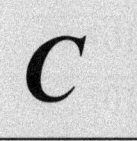

BURIAL FUND	100, 111
BUY-IN PROGRAMS, COVERAGE	95, 109

C

CATEGORICALLY NEEDY	96, 106
CO-PAYMENTS/DEDUCTIBLES	95, 109
COUNTABLE INCOME	98, 111
Earned income	98
In-kind income	99
Unearned income	98-99

Topical Index (TI)
Medicaid
(continued)

COUNTABLE RESOURCES	99
Continuing care retirement community entrance fee	99
Defined	99
Home equity	99

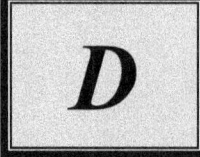

DEEMING OF INCOME AND RESOURCES	100
DUAL ELIGIBLES	109-110

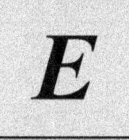

ELIGIBILTY FACTORS	
Categories of eligibles	96, 106-108
Income and resources	98-99, 114
Residence in SSI and Section 209(b) states	96, 106-107, 114
Status	98
ELIGIBILITY REQUIREMENTS, CATEGORICAL	
Age	98, 107
Disability or blindness	97, 107
SSI recipients	98, 114
ELIGIBILITY REQUIREMENTS, NON-FINANCIAL	
Citizenship	96, 98
Residency	96
EXEMPT RESOURCES (see Resources, exempt)	
EXEMPT TRUSTS	
Income-only trust	114

Long-term Care at Home Consumer Guide   292   © 2009 Walter Feldesman

Miller trust	108, 113
Pooled trust	113-114
Trust for disabled persons under age 65	109

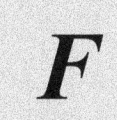

FAMILY ALLOWANCE	102, 103, 105

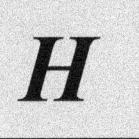

HOME HEALTH SERVICES	
Conditions to obtaining	124
Services included	122-123
HOMESTEAD	
Countable (non-countable resource)	99, 118
Excess shelter allowance	102-103
Lien on	127
Transfer of	119

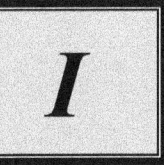

INCOME (see also Countable income)	
Actual availability	98
Definition of	98
In-kind support	99
INSTITUTIONALIZED PERSONS	
Allocation of income between community spouse and	100
Asset transfers	118-119

Topical Index (TI)
Medicaid
(continued)

Defined	100
Personal needs allowance	105-106
Spouse of (community spouse)	100

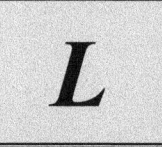

LONG-TERM CARE INSURANCE PARTNERSHIP PROGRAMS	134-135
LOW-INCOME MEDICARE BENEFICIARIES	
Deductibles, coinsurance, co-payments, premiums, payment by Medicaid	95, 109
Dual eligibles, defined	109-110
Income/resource guidelines for QMB beneficiaries	109
Qualified disabled/working individual income (QDWI), resource limits for payment of Part A premiums	111-111
Low-income qualifying individual (QI-1), income/resource limits	110
Qualified Medicare beneficiary (QMB), buy-in to Medicare by Medicaid	109-110
Specified low-income Medicare beneficiary (SLMB), income/resource limits	110

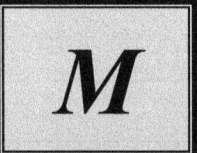

MAXIMUM AND MINIMUM COMMUNITY SPOUSE RESOURCE ALLOWANCE (Spousal Impoverishment)	
Generally	102-104
Assessment of couples' resources	101-102, 104
Community spouse, amount of resources allowed to keep	103-104

Topical Index (TI)
Medicaid
(continued)

Deeming procedures	101
Duration of institutionalization, thirty (30) days minimum requirement	101-102, 104
Excessive spousal resources, contribution to cost of institutionalized care	104
Federal law, maximum amount of spousal resources allowed under	103-104
Institutionalized spouse, transfer of resources to community spouse	102, 105
Minimum monthly income allowance, duty of states to provide	102
Permitted deductions	105
Personal needs allowance, amount under Medicaid program	105-106
Snapshot rule	102
MEDICAID	
Generally	95
Buy-in programs	95, 109-110
Joint Federal-state program	95
Means-tested program	95, 96
Optional services	122, 124-126
Medically oriented	122-123, 124
Non-medically oriented	122-123
Waivered services	122-123
MEDICALLY NEEDY	
Generally	107
Medically need income level	96, 107
Services covered	107
Spend down options	96, 98, 107

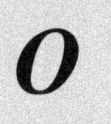

OPTIONAL CATEGORICALLY NEEDY	
Absolute dollar cap	108
Income cap states	107-108, 114
Resource standards	108
Services covered	108
300% program	108, 114

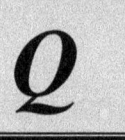

PERSONAL CARE SERVICES	
Application for	125
Basic requirements for provision of	125
Fiscal assessment	125
Nursing assessment	125
Personal care, defined	123
Services defined	123
Social assessment	125
PERSONAL NEEDS ALLOWANCE	105-106

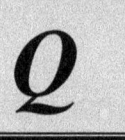

QUALIFIED DISABLED AND WORKING INDIVIDUALS	
Poverty level needed to qualify	75

Premium payment through Medicaid/Medicare	75
QUALIFIED MEDICARE BENEFICIARIES	
Generally	74, 109
Premium payments	109
Social Security cost-of-living increases, effect of	74
Subsets of	75
Dual eligibles	74
Low-income qualifying individual (QI-1)	75
Specified low-income Medicare beneficiary (SLMB)	74-75
Qualified disabled and working individual	75

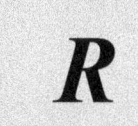

RECOVERY BY MEDICAID	
Community spouse	127-128
Estate of Medicaid recipient	127-128
RESIDENCY REQUIREMENT	35, 96
RESOURCES (see also Countable resources)	
Definition of	99
Joint bank accounts	99
Maximum/minimum community spouse resource allowance	103
Retirement funds	99
Spousal	100, 104
RESOURCES, EXEMPT	
Automobile	100
Burial plot and funds	100
Homestead	99
Life insurance	100

Personal property	100

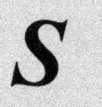

SERVICES COVERED BY MEDICAID (see Medicaid; Home health care services)	
SPECIAL NEEDS TRUST (Supplemental needs trust)	112
SPECIFIED LOW-INCOME MEDICARE BENEFICIARY (SLMB)	102-103, 105
SPOUSAL BUDGETING	
Community spouse, description of	100-105, 108
income allowance	102
refusal to contribute	101
resource allowance	102-104
Family allowance	102-103, 105
Institutionalized spouse	102, 106
assignment of right to support	104-105
income allowance (see personal needs allowance)	
Resources	100
Snapshot rule	101-102
Spousal refusal	101, 104
SURPLUS INCOME AND RESOURCES (see spend down)	104

T

TRANSFER OF ASSETS	
Civil penalties for wrongful transfer of assets	115, 117
Exemptions from transfer penalty rule	115, 118
Fair market value, penalty for transferring assets under	117
Ineligibility period	115, 117-118
Irrevocable Miller Trust, exclusion	119-120
Irrevocable trust, degree subjected to trust transfer rules	119
Look-back period	115, 117
Medicare services subject to transfer penalties	120-121
Pooled trust, disabled person(s) excluded from	119-120
Revocable trust, exclusion from trust transfer rule	119
Transfer penalty (civil)	117
Trust for disabled persons, exemption from trust transfer rules	119
TRUST ELIBILITY RULES	
Exempt trusts	112
Irrevocable living trust	111-112
Living revocable (*inter vivos*) trust	111
Special/supplemental needs trust, defined	1112
Testamentary trust	111
Third-party grantor trust, defined	112

Topical Index (TI)
Medicaid
(continued)

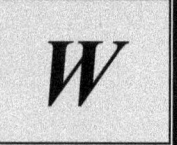

WAIVERED SERVICES	
Home and community-based long-term care	122-123

TOPICAL INDEX

Medicare Outpatient Prescription Drugs

(References are to pages in Chapter 5)

A

Alternative prescription drug coverage	137, 145-46
Appeals	139
Automatic enrollment, none (Medicare Part D)	137 140
Automatically eligible (Part D)	141

B

Benefits, standard drug plan	139
Brand-name drugs (Medicare Part D)	140, 153, 154

C

Catastrophic coverage	145
Changes to plan	139, 142
Co-payment, coinsurance (Medicare Part D)	137, 145-147, 152-154
Continuous period of eligibility (Medicare Part D)	141
Cost-sharing (Medicare Part D)	137, 143, 145-147, 153
Covered drugs	139
Creditable coverage	142-144

**Topical Index (TI)
Medicare Outpatient Prescription Drugs
(continued)**

D

Deductible (Medicare Part D)	137, 145-147, 149, 151
Doughnut hole	145-147, 152-153
Drug-only plan (Medicare Part D)	141
Dual eligibles (Medicare Part D)	141-143

E

Eligibility (Medicare Part D)	140
Employer-sponsored drug benefit programs	140, 144
End-stage renal disease (ESRD)	140
Enhanced alternative coverage	146
Enrollment	137, 140-142
Expedited coverage determination	139
Extra help subsidy	137, 147-148

F

Formulary	139, 143
Full-benefit dual eligible (Medicare Part D)	142-143, 151-153
Full-subsidy eligible individual (Medicare Part D)	151-153

G

Generic drug	130, 146, 153-154

Topical Index (TI)
Medicare Outpatient Prescription Drugs
(continued)

Generic drug co-payment amount	153-154

I

Initial coverage limit	144-145, 152
Initial enrollment period (Medicare Part D)	141
Institutionalized dual eligibles, non-payment of deductibles based on	154

L

Late enrollment, premium penalty based on	143-144
Late filing penalty/surcharge (Medicare Part D)	143-144
Low-income Part D subsidy for low-income individuals	151
Low-income Part D subsidy for full-benefit dual eligibles	151

M

Medicaid, as relates to Medicare Part D	138
Medicare Advantage Prescription Drug Plans (MA-PDPs)	140-141
Medicare Part D	140
Medicare Prescription Drug Improvement and Modernization Act (MMA) (*see* also Medicare Part D)	137
Medicare Prescription Drug Program	137
Medigap insurance policies, prohibited use after 1/1/2006	138
Monthly drug premium, standard drug benefit	145

N

Non-formulary drug	139

Topical Index (TI)
Medicare Outpatient Prescription Drugs
(continued)

O

Out-of-pocket expenses	145-146, 152
Out-of-pocket threshold (Medicare Part D)	145-146, 153-154
Outpatient prescription drugs (Medicare Part D)	141
Overview	137-139

P

Part D-eligible individuals	137
Partial-subsidy eligible individuals	151-153
Periods of enrollment	141-141
Poverty level, effect on payment for drug discount care	151-153
Premium (Medicare Part D)	146-147
Premium subsidy	147, 152-153
Prescription drugs (Original Medicare)	140
Prescription drugs (Medicare Part D)	137
Prior 2006 Medigap policies covering drugs, continued use of	138

Q

Qualified Medicare beneficiary	152
Qualified prescription drug coverage	137
Qualifying individual (QI-1)	152

S

Special enrollment period (Medicare Part D)	141-142

Topical Index (TI)
Medicare Outpatient Prescription Drugs
(continued)

Specified low-income Medicare beneficiary (SLMB)	152
Stand-alone prescription drug plans	137, 140-141, 144
Standard coverage determination	139
Standard drug plan	145-146
Subsidy-eligible individual	140, 147, 151
Subsidies (see Extra help)	

Topical Index (TI)
Medicare Advantage Plans
(continued)

TOPICAL INDEX

Medicare Advantage Plans

(References are to pages in Chapter 6)

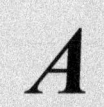

ACCESS TO SERVICE	
Choice of primary care physician	163, 180
Emergency service requirements	164-165
Initial assessment	181
Prompt/continued service, necessity for	181
Requirement of private fee-for-service plan	172
Specialty care, access to required of coordinated care plans	163-164, 181
ANNUAL COORDINATED ELECTION PERIOD	
Annual election selection, month of year to be made	155, 158-159, 161
Change of election	155, 157, 158
Freedom of selection during election period	159
APPEALS	
ALJ hearing	176
Departmental Appeals Board review	176
Grievances	167-170
Fast-track appeals	166, 177
Organization determinations, standard and expedited	170-172
Reconsideration determinations, standard and expedited	173-175

B

BALANCED BUDGET ACT OF 1997 (BBA) – MEDICARE+CHOICE PROGRAM	
Impact of BBA on Medicare program	165
Medicare + Choice replaced by Medicare Advantage	165
BENEFITS	
Additional benefits	162-163
Basic benefits, types enrollees entitled to	161
Non-MSA plans, rules for participating in optional supplemental benefits, explained	162-163
Supplemental benefits, mandatory purchase under a MSA plan	162

C

CAPITATION	
Defined and explained	183
Medicare Advantage capitation payments	162, 183, 185, 200-201, 204
Coordinated care plans (See also Medicare Advantage Coordinated Care Plans, this index)	153, 176

E

ELECTION OF PLANS (ENROLLMENT)	
Generally	158-159
Annual coordination of election period	155, 159

Beneficiary, freedom to choose plan during annual coordinated election period	155, 158
Beneficiary's moving, continuation of special enrollment period thereafter	159
Change of election, time for making change	158-159
Disenrollment period	159
Election periods	158-159
Enrollment/disenrollment, coordination by organizations	158-159
Enrollment in Medical Savings Account, special rules	160-161, 197
Initial enrollment	158
Open enrollment period	159
Special enrollment periods	159
Termination of plan	158, 160
ELECTION PERIODS (See Election of plans)	
ELIGIBILITY	
Medical Savings Accounts	196-197
Specialized Medicare Advantage plans for special needs beneficiaries	194
EMERGENCY SERVICES	
Emergency services, defined	164
Prudent lay person test, application at	165
Enrolment (See Election of plans, this index)	158-161

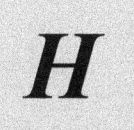

HEALTH MAINTENANCE ORGANIZATION (HMO) (See Medicare Advantage Health Maintenance Organization, this index)	

Topical Index (TI)
Medicare Advantage Plans
(continued)

I

INITIAL ENROLLMENT (See Election of plans, this index)	

L

LICENSED UNDER STATE LAW	
MA organizations, required licensed by state	182, 185, 188
Provider-sponsored organizations (PSO), exemption from state license requirement	189
Regional Fraternal Benefits (RFB) plans, requirements for state license	192
LOCAL PREFERRED PROVIDER ORGANIZATIONS (See Medicare Advantage Regional Preferred Provider Organizations, this index)	

M

MA PLANS PART D COVERAGE	
Coordinated care plan, mandatory drug coverage under	156
Fee-for-service plans, choice to offer Part D coverage	206
MEDICAL SAVINGS PLAN (See Medicare Advantage Medical Savings Account Plans, this index)	
MEDICARE ADVANTAGE (MA) COORDINATED CARE PLANS	
Generally	180
Categories of MA plans	157, 180

Topical Index (TI)
Medicare Advantage Plans
(continued)

Charge limits (Balance billing) involving non-contract providers	158, 180
Charge limits (Balance billing) involving providers under contract	181-182
Coordinated care plans, flexibility/choice between	182
Initial assessment of health needs requirements	163, 181
MA coordinated care plan, defined	180
Network of appropriate providers, need to maintain	180
Operating "around the clock," requirement pertaining to	164, 181
Premiums, not required to cover Medicare basic benefits	161, 181
Primary care physician (PCP) panel, establishment of	163, 180
Specialty (specialist) care, need to provide access to	163-164, 181
MEDICARE ADVANTAGE HEALTH MAINTENANCE ORGANIZATION (HMO)	
HMO, defined	183
Limit of enrollee's financial liability	184
Lock-in features in HMO provider cases, explained	183
Point of service, optional benefit offered by HMOs	184
Primary care physician, need to choose	183
Specialist, need to obtain referral from primary care physician	183
MEDICARE ADVANTAGE MEDICAL SAVINGS ACCOUNT (MSA) PLANS	
Annual deductible payment requirements	198
BBA of 1997, MSA plan established under	196
Choice of health professionals	199
Commingling funds, prohibition against	199
Contract-bound physician, Medicare payment as full payment	201

Eligibility requirements	196-197
Enrollment procedures into MSA program	160-161, 197
High-deductible features of a MSA	197-198
HIPAA of 1996, MSAs established under	196
Income from MSA accounts, tax treatment	201-203
Medicare as sole contributor to MSA	200
Medigap/other policies, prohibition against sales of	200
MSA tax exclusion provisions	198
Physician's charges, limitations on in MSA program	201
Premium charges, absence of limits on	200
Qualified medical expense, defined	198
Tax treatment of MSAs	201-202
MEDICARE ADVANTAGE PREFERRED PROVIDER (PPO) ORGANIZATION PLANS	
Limits on enrollee's liability	185
Local and regional PPOs (See in this index, Medicare Advantage regional PPO plans)	186
PPO, defined	185
State licensure requirements, need to comply with	185
Unlicensed PPO, partnership with state-licensed carrier	185
MEDICARE PRIVATE FEE-FOR-SERVICE (PFFS) PLANS	
Defined	204
Contracting physicians, restrictions on fees charged by	205
Medicare fee restrictions on PFFS claims	205

Topical Index (TI)
Medicare Advantage Plans
(continued)

Notice to enrollees by hospital, requirements for	206
Part D drug coverage, optional for PFFS plans	206
Premiums, absence of limits on	204
Prescription drug coverage	206
Quality assurance, no requirement for	206
MEDICARE ADVANTAGE PROGRAM	
Generally	155
Annual election plan switching provision	159
Compared to Original Medicare	155-156
Types of plans	157-158
MEDICARE ADVANTAGE PROVIDER-SPONSORED ORGANIZATION (PSO)	
Minimum number of enrollees rule	189
PSO, defined	189
Overview of PSO program	189
Payment limitation on physician's charges	190
Services to enrollees, minimum under Part A, Part B rules	190
State licensure requirements	189
MEDICARE ADVANTAGE RELIGIOUS FRATERNAL BENEFIT (RFB) PLANS	
Church membership requirement under RFB Plan	192
Professional health network requirement	192
RFB plan, defined	191
RFB state licensure requirements	192
MEDICARE ADVANTAGE SPECIALIZED PLANS FOR SPECIAL NEEDS BENEFICIARIES (SNP)	
Case-by-case determination of need	193

Topical Index (TI)
Medicare Advantage Plans
(continued)

Disproportionate percentage SNP, defined	193
Eligibility requirements under SNP	194
"Grandfathered" beneficiaries, distinguished	194
Ineligibility of beneficiary, deeming based on meeting criteria	194
Part D drug coverage, SNPs required to provide	193
Special needs individual, defined	193
MEDICARE+CHOICE (NOW MEDICARE ADVANTAGE) PROGRAM	
BBA of 1997, establishment of M+C under	155
Part A, Part B eligibles coverage under M+C program	155
Types of M+C Plans	157-158
MEDICARE SECONDARY PAYER PROVISIONS	
MA organizations, right to seek payment from primary payer	164
Medicare's right to seek recovery from primary payer	164
Recovery of incorrect payments, three-year limitation pertaining to	164

O

OPEN ENROLLMENT AND DISENROLLMENT PERIODS (See Election of Plans (Enrollment), this index)	

P

PREMIUMS	
Coordinated care plans, no premiums charged for Medicare	161

Topical Index (TI)
Medicare Advantage Plans
(continued)

basic benefits	
Limitations on premiums charged	161
Monthly basic premiums, methodology used for calculating	161
Monthly supplemental premiums, basis for charging	161
Unlimited premiums, MSA and PFFS plans allowed to charge	158, 161
PRIVATE FEE-FOR-SERVICE (PFFS) PLANS (See Medicare Advantage Private Fee-for-Service Plans)	

S

SPECIAL ELECTION PERIOD (See Election of Plans (Enrollment), this index)	
SPECIAL RULES FOR ENROLLING IN A MSA (See Election of Plans (Enrollment), this index)	

TOPICAL INDEX

Medicare Advantage Outpatient Drugs
(References are to pages in Chapter 7)

A

Alternative prescription drug coverage	210
Automatic enrollment	212

B

Benefits, alternative prescription drug plan	210
Benefits, standard drug plan	208-210
Brand-name drugs	209, 212, 220-221

C

Catastrophic coverage	209
Changes to plan	215
Coinsurance, co-payment, cost-sharing	209, 211, 220-222
Cost-sharing	208, 210-211, 220-222
Covered drugs	207

D

Deductible	207, 209-211, 220-222

**Topical Index (TI)
Medicare Advantage Outpatient Drugs
(continued)**

Doughnut hole	209-210, 220-221
Drug-only plan	211
Dual eligibles	208, 212, 216-217, 221

E

Eligibility/election date enrollment	213-215
Enhanced alternative coverage	210
Enrollment	212-215
End-stage renal disease (ESRD)	211
Expedited coverage determination	208
Extra-help subsidy	211

F

Formulary coverage, appeals concerning	207-208
Full-benefit dual eligible	216-217, 218-219
Full-subsidy eligible individual	218-221

G

Generic drug	220-222

I

Initial coverage limit	208-209
Initial enrollment period	213

Topical Index (TI)
Medicare Advantage Outpatient Drugs
(continued)

Involuntary disenrollment	215

L

Late enrollment, premium penalty based on	216
Low-income premium subsidy	219-220
Low-income subsidy individual	218

M

Medicaid, as relates to Medicare Part D	208
Medicare Prescription Drug Improvement and Modernization Act (MMA) (*see* also Medicare Part D)	207
Medicare private fee-for-service (PFFS) plans	217
Medigap insurance policies, prohibited use of drug coverage after 1/1/2006	208

O

Out-of-pocket expenses	209-210, 220
Out-of-pocket threshold	209-210, 220-222
Outpatient prescription drugs	207-208, 213

P

Part D-eligible individuals	208-210, 212-213, 218
Partial-subsidy-eligible individuals	218, 221-222
Periods of enrollment	213-214
Poverty level, effect on payment for drug discount care	218-219

Topical Index (TI)
Medicare Advantage Outpatient Drugs
(continued)

Premium	208-209, 211
Premium subsidy	217, 219-220
Prescription drug plans	207, 212-213
Prior 2006 Medigap policies covering drugs, continued use of	208

S

Special enrollment period	213-214
Specified low-income Medicare beneficiary (SLMB)	216, 219
Standard coverage determination	208
Standard drug coverage	208-210
Subsidy eligible individual	218
Subsidies, extra help	211, 220

T

Termination of plan	215

TOPICAL INDEX

Private Payment for Care
(References are to pages in Chapters 8-16)

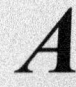

ACCELERATION OF LIFE INSURANCE BENEFITS (Chapter 12)	
Chronically-ill persons in viatical settlement cases	255
Qualified long-term care life insurance contracts	255-256
Qualified long-term services, defined	256
Tax status of accelerated life insurance benefits	256
Terminally-ill person in viatical settlement cases	256
Viatical settlement, explained	255, 258
ADULT DAY CARE CENTERS (Chapter 13)	
National Adult Day Care Service Association, levels of care prescribed by	259
Attendance, effect on homebound status	248
Days-of-week coverage	260
Generally	259
Payment for adult day care services	260
Types of adult day care programs	259
ANNUITIES (Chapter 14)	
Immediate annuity, defined	261
Deferred annuity, defined	261
Fixed annuity, defined	261

Topical Index (TI)
Private Payment for Care
(continued)

Generally	261
Joint survivor annuity, defined	261
Single life annuity, defined	261
Tax assessed in annuity cases	262
Variable annuity, defined	261

C

CHOOSING HOUSING ALTERNATIVES (Chapter 15)	
Accessory unit	267
Assisted living costs, methods of payment	264
Assisted living facility, services performed in	264
Cluster care	267
Congregate housing	267-268
Continuing care retirement community (CCRC), described	265-266
Elder cottage housing opportunity (ECHO) unit	267-269
Generally	251-252
Independent living retirement community, described	266-267
Naturally occurring retirement community (NORC)	263-265
Non-medical facilities for dependent residents, list of	264-265
Non-institutional/non-medical facilities, list of	265
Shared housing	269
Types of CCRC contracts	266
Extensive contract	266
Fee-for service continuing care contract	266
Modified fee-for-service contract	266

H

HOME EQUITY CONVERSION PLAN: REVERSE MORTGAGE (Chapter 11)

Generally	251-252
Reverse mortgage, explained	251-252
Sale-leaseback, explained	251

L

LONG-TERM CARE INSURANCE (LTCI) (Chapter 9)

Benefits derived from LTCI	240-241
Change in premium level, state approval required	239
Characteristics of LTCI policies	237-238
Cognitive impairment trigger	238
Daily activity of living trigger	238-239
Generally	235, 237
Home care coverage	224
Indemnity nature of LTCI policies	235
Inflation protection, availability of	241, 244-245
Medical necessity trigger	238
Non-forfeiture clause	240, 242-243
Pre-existing condition	242
Premium costs for LTCI policies, factors affecting	239
Premium level, stabilizing provisions	239
State Partnership Program (Robert Wood Johnson Program)	246

Topical Index (TI)
Private Payment for Care
(continued)

Tax advantage for tax-qualified LTCI policies	245-247
Tax-qualified LTCI policy, qualifying conditions	243-244
Triggers, commencement of coverage based on	238-239
Types Of LTCI policies issued	
Classic policy	237
Integrated policy	237
Unintentional lapse of LTCI policy, reinstatement provision	243
Upgrading LTCI policies, procedures to be followed	242
Waiting period, elimination of	241-242
Waiver of premiums on LTCI policy based on length of time	240

M

MEDICARE SUPPLEMENTAL INSURANCE (MEDIGAP) (Chapter 8)	
Age 65 and over, enrollment in Medigap without pre-existing condition exclusion	225, 232
Annual out-of-pocket expenses, payment under high-deductible plan	223, 229
Attained age, method for establishing premium	226
Availability of Medigap policies	223
Benefits	
Additional benefits contained in Plans B-J	227-228
Basic benefits contained in Plan A	225, 227
Summary of benefits (chart)	233-234
BBA of 1997, changes made to Medigap policies by	223
Characteristics of Medigap policies	223, 230

Community rating, method for establishing premium	226
Creditable coverage	225, 231
Free look of 30 days afforded to applicant	225
Guaranteed issue of Medigap policy in spite of pre-existing condition	225, 231-232
High-deductible policies	
Amount of deductible	229
Description of, Plans H and J	223, 229
Home care coverage	230
Issue age, method for establishing premium	226
Medicare Select	223-224, 229-230
Open enrollment period	225, 230, 231
Plans K and L	223, 228-229
Portability	226
Pre-existing conditions, waiver of waiting period under BBA of 1997	225, 231-232
Premiums	208, 211
Prescription drug coverage, not allowed after January 1, 2006	229
Standardized plans, twelve (12)	223
Ten standard Medigap policies, designated in 1992	223

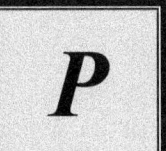

PRIVATE PAYMENT TO PROVIDERS OF HOME CARE (Chapter 10)	
Direct contracting	247-248
Processing care through home health agency	248

Topical Index (TI)
Private Payment for Care
(continued)

Geriatric care managers (case management)	249-250

Word Index

This index lists the most significant words and terms used in the *Guide*. Where reference is made to multiple pages, the reader can quickly identify the particular chapter where the word or term appears by consulting the table below.

Chapter 1	Introduction to Home Care – Home Care Basics	1-15
Chapter 2	Where to Obtain Home Care	17-29
Chapter 3	Original Medicare (Parts A/B) – A Federal Source of Payment	31-93
Chapter 4	Medicaid – A Federal and State Source of Payment	95-135
Chapter 5	Original Medicare Prescription Drugs (Part D)	137-154
Chapter 6	Medicare Advantage Plans (MAP) – A Federal Source of Payment	155-206
Chapter 7	Medicare Advantage Outpatient Prescription Drug Plans (MA-PDP)	207-222
Chapter 8	Medicare Supplemental Insurance (Medigap)	223-234
Chapter 9	Private Long-term Care Insurance	235-246
Chapter 10	Private Payment for Home Care	247-250
Chapter 11	Using a Home to Pay for Home Care	251-254
Chapter 12	Accelerated Benefits of a Life Insurance Policy to Pay for Home Care	255-258
Chapter 13	Use of Adult Day Care Centers for Eldercare Outside the Home	259-260
Chapter 14	Use of Annuities to Pay for Eldercare	261-262
Chapter 15	Alternative Housing Facilities – Private Payment	263-269
Chapter 16	Federal Housing and Subsidies	271-274

Word Index (WI)
(continued)

WORD INDEX (WI)

(References are to pages)

A

Abdominal aorta aneurism screening	90
Accelerated benefits	255-257
Accessory unit	265, 267
Activities of daily living (ADL)	1, 26, 49, 121, 237-239, 244, 255, 259, 264
Actual charge	73, 93
Acute care	2
Acupuncture	70
Additional benefits	161-163, 225, 227
Additional out-of-pocket expenses (for drugs)	145, 146, 209, 210
Additional services	161-163, 204, 265
Administration on Aging	28
Administrative law judge (ALJ)	56-57, 168, 173, 176, 178
Administrative law judge hearing	168, 173, 176
Adult day care center	2, 15, 25-27, 60, 237, 259-260
Adult home	154, 221, 263
Advance directive	20
Aliens (see also Permanent resident alien)	35, 96
Alternative prescription drug plan coverage (Part D)	137, 145-146, 208, 210

Word Index (WI)
(continued)

Alzheimer's disease	25, 90, 239, 249
Ambulance transportation	66, 87
Amyotrophic lateral sclerosis	35
Annual deposit (Medical Savings Account)	197-198, 200
Annuity	117, 128, 261-262, 251-252
Ankle-brachial test	90
Annual coordinated election period	141, 155, 159, 161, 213
Annual deductible	68, 78, 82, 88, 137, 145-146, 162, 198, 200, 202, 210, 227
Annual enrollment	143, 159
Appeals	20, 55-56, 129, 131, 139, 167-174, 207
Appliances	52
Applicant spouse (Medicaid)	100, 101
Application	32, 35, 37-40, 61, 101-102, 105, 115-117, 125-126, 129, 137, 149, 188, 230, 242
Application for enrollment	35, 38
Application for personal care	125
Approved charge	47, 68, 71, 73, 78, 82, 165, 227
Area agency on aging	17, 28-29
Artificial eyes, limbs	66
Assessment of resources (Snapshot Rule)	101-102

Long-term Care at Home Consumer Guide   329   © 2009 Walter Feldesman

Word Index (WI)
(continued)

Assets	77, 99, 102, 106, 109, 111-113, 115-121, 127-128, 134, 187, 199, 202, 246, 251, 272-273
Assignment	47, 68, 72-73, 104, 216, 258
Assisted living facilities/program	154, 221, 250, 263-265, 272
Attained age	35, 226
Attendants	1, 7, 22, 123-124, 247
Automatic enrollment (Eligibility)	37, 119, 141, 212
Average cost of nursing facility care	118

B

Balance billing (see also Charge limit)	73, 91, 158, 163, 166, 181, 205-206
Balanced Budget Act of 1997	60, 81, 96, 130, 165, 196, 223, 229, 230-231
Basic allowance	102-103
Basic beneficiary premium	161
Basic benefits (Medicare)	157, 158, 161-162, 166, 170, 185, 190, 200-201, 204, 227
Bathing	1, 7, 45, 49, 123, 228, 230, 239, 244, 249
Benchmark plan	221

Bidding methodology	195
Billing (see also Balance billing)	55, 72-73, 92, 158, 165, 205
Biologicals	45, 48, 52, 81, 85
Blind	25, 96, 98, 106, 114, 119
Blood-clotting factors	66
Blood glucose monitor	67
Blood transfusions	81
Board-and-care home	1, 263, 267
Bone mass measurement	68
Braces	66, 83
Brand-name drug (Medicare Part D)	140, 153, 154, 209, 212, 221-222
Breast cancer screening	88
Burial expenses	100, 111
Burial fund	100
Buy-in	74, 95, 109, 152, 219

C

Cane	47, 83
Capitation	61, 162, 183, 185, 198, 200-201, 204
Cardiovascular screening blood tests	88
Carrier	24, 32, 70, 72, 185, 189, 226, 242

Word Index (WI)
(continued)

Carve-out coverage	63, 93
Case management	24, 49, 60, 123, 130, 132, 133
Casts	66, 81
Cataract surgery	68
Catheters	48
Catastrophic coverage (Part D)	145, 209
Catastrophic limits	187
Categorically needy	96, 106-107
Center for Health Dispute Resolution	176
Centers for Medicare and Medicaid Services (CMS) (see also Health Care Financing Administration)	31-32, 35, 38, 61, 70, 81, 90, 114, 130, 139, 142, 149, 158, 160, 163, 168, 173, 175, 180-181, 185, 187-188, 193-194, 198, 205, 207, 212, 215, 217, 219, 230
Certificate of medical necessity	84-85, 87
Certified home health agency (CHHA)	10, 18, 19-20, 41, 45, 54, 122, 124, 248
Change of election	159
Charge limit (see also Balance billing; Limiting charge)	79, 91, 165, 181, 190, 201, 205
Chiropractor's services	65
Chronic care (long-term care)	2
Chronic condition	193, 235
Claim determination	55

Word Index (WI)
(continued)

Clean claim	171
Clinical laboratory tests	90
Cluster care	267
Coinsurance (see also Co-payments; Deductibles)	47, 61, 67-68, 71 73-74, 81, 88-89, 93, 109, 137, 145, 154, 156, 161, 184, 185, 194, 209, 222-223, 227, 233, 243-244, 255
Cognitive impairment trigger	238
Colonoscopy	89
Colorectal cancer screening	89
Colostomy care	43
Community-based agencies	24
Community-based services	49
Community-based waiver services	104
Community mental health center	82
Community spouse	100, 102-105, 108, 111, 117, 127
Community spouse excess resources	101
Community spouse income allowance	102-103
Community spouse refusal	101, 104, 127
Community spouse resource allowance	103-104
Comprehensive outpatient rehabilitation facility	68, 77, 82, 177
Conditions of participation	10, 18, 248
Confinement to the home	1, 6
Congregate housing	267-268, 267, 274

Word Index (WI)
(continued)

Congregate meals program	14, 29, 49
Consolidated Omnibus Budget Reconciliation Act (COBRA)	33, 64, 108, 134, 199
Continuation insurance	184
Continued eligibility	194
Continuing care retirement community	101, 265
Continuous period of institutionalization	101-102, 104
Cooking	1, 46, 249, 269
Coordination of coverage, Medicare and employer plans	33, 63, 93
Coordinated care plan	157, 161-163, 166, 179, 180-178, 179, 181, 186, 189, 191-193
Co-payment (see also Deductibles; Coinsurance)	36, 49, 52, 61, 71, 73, 78, 81, 95, 109, 145-147, 151, 153-156, 161-162, 184, 198, 205, 209-211, 218, 220-224, 230, 233
Cosmetic surgery	69
Cost-basis HMO	217, 231, 232
Cost-sharing	61, 71, 93, 131, 139, 142, 145-147, 151-152, 153-154, 155-156, 161-162, 185, 196, 208, 210-211, 218, 220-222, 228
Cost-sharing subsidies	220

Word Index (WI)
(continued)

Counseling	19, 46, 52, 90, 245 253-254
Countable income	98-99, 107, 111-112
Countable resources	99, 104, 107, 111
Covered dugs (Part D)	139, 209
Coverage gap (for drugs) (see also Doughnut hole)	145-147, 209-211
Creditable coverage	142, 144, 214, 216, 225, 231
Critical access hospital	87
Crutches	83
Custodial account	198
Custodial care	2, 4, 7-8, 69, 121, 235, 264

D

Deductibles and co-payments (see also Coinsurance; Co-payment; Annual deductible)	36, 49, 52, 61, 67-68, 71, 73-74, 78, 81-82, 88-90, 93, 95, 109, 145-147, 151-154, 156, 161-163, 184-187, 192, 197-198, 205, 208-211, 218, 220-224, 227-230, 233, 239, 241, 243-244, 255
Deeming	100-101
Deferred annuity	261

Word Index (WI)
(continued)

Deficit Reduction Act	134, 246
Demand billing	55
Denial (benefits)	105, 129, 139, 167
Dental services/care	70, 85, 93, 122, 155-156, 161, 199-200
Department of Health and Human Services (HHS)	25, 31, 95
Departmental appeals board	168, 176, 178
Dependents	34-35, 102, 199, 202-203
Dependent services (Home care)	1, 7, 41, 44
Designated services	118, 119, 121
Determinations	32, 54, 56, 139, 167-177
Diabetes	67, 88-89
Diagnostic tests /services	68, 90
Dialysis	34, 43, 67-68, 87, 170
Digital rectal exam	88
Direct contracting	2, 12, 15, 247-249
Disability	12, 28, 31, 37, 75, 107, 110, 200, 244, 247
Disability benefits	34-35, 272
Disabled individuals	i, 95, 120
Discharge of patients	8, 23
Discharge planners	2
Disenrollment	159-160, 215
Dishwashing	46

Word Index (WI)
(continued)

Disproportionate (Specialized needs plan)	193-194
Disruptive behavior	215
Domiciliary care home	263
Doughnut hole	145-147, 152-153, 209-210, 220-221
Dressing	1, 7, 45, 80, 123, 228, 230, 239, 244
Dressing changes	7, 43, 45
Drug-only plan (Medicare Part D)	141, 213
Drugs (Original Medicare)	66-67, 81, 137
Drugs (Medicare Part D)	137, 139-141, 144-147, 149, 151, 153, 155
Dual eligibles	36, 74, 109, 130, 141-143, 208, 212, 216-217, 221
Durable medical equipment	45, 47, 49

E

Eating	1, 7, 228, 230, 244
Ear ailments	65
Earned income	98
Efficiency assessment	125
Elder cottage housing opportunity (ECHO) unit	267-268
Electronic beeper system	8
Eligibility (Original Medicare)	32, 34, 51
Eligibility (Medicare Part D)	140

Word Index (WI)
(continued)

Eligibility factors	18, 31, 41-42
Eligibility for persons age 65 or older (see Enrollment)	28, 35, 37-38
Emergency care	131, 228
Emergency hospital care	32, 44, 69, 79, 81, 91
Emergency medical condition	69, 131, 164-165
Emergency response system	8, 13, 121
Emergency services	131, 164-165, 170, 224, 230
Emergency services based on a prudent lay-person test	164-165
Employee's election under employer health plan	64
Employer group health plan	34, 39, 63, 70, 157
End-stage renal disease (ESRD)	34, 87, 140, 155-157, 194, 196, 211
Enhanced alternative coverage	146, 210
Enrollee-provider communications	132
Enrollment (Medicaid managed care)	129-132
Enrollment (Medical Savings Account)	197
Enrollment (Medicare Advantage plan)	157, 158-160, 193, 212
Enrollment (Original Medicare)	35, 37-40, 64, 74
Enrollment (Part D)	137, 140-142, 143, 212
Enrollment periods	38, 39, 141-143, 158, 213-215
Enrollment requirements and limitations	37-40
Equipment (see also Durable medical equipment)	4, 19, 45, 47, 67, 83-85, 87, 100, 249

Exception to formulary (Part D)	139, 207
Excess shelter allowance	102, 103, 105
Exclusion coverage	63, 93
Exclusion ratio	262
Exclusions (Medicare Part B)	69-70
Exempt resources	99, 101
Exempt transfers	74
Exempt trusts	112, 115, 118, 120
Expedited coverage determination (Part D)	139, 208
Expedited grievance	55, 58, 169
Expedited organization determination	58, 171-172
Expedited reconsideration determination	58-59, 174-175
Expedited time frame	139, 171
Expenses in calculating spend down	107-108, 114
Explanation of medical benefits	206
Extra help subsidy	137, 147-148, 211
Eyeglasses	66, 68, 70, 86, 161

F

Facility discharge planner	8
Fair hearing	103, 129
False teeth	66, 199
Family allowance	102-103, 105
Fast-track appeals	177-178
Fecal-occult blood test	89

Word Index (WI)
(continued)

Federal Employee Health Benefits Program	197
Federal poverty level	74-75, 102, 109-110, 151-153, 154, 218-222
Fee schedule	85, 182, 201, 205
Feeding	19, 43, 45, 49, 123, 239
Fiscal assessment	125
Fiscal intermediary	54, 55, 56
Fixed annuity	261
Flat monthly maintenance allowance	103
Flexible sigmoidoscopy	89
Flu shot	67
Foot care	50, 65, 69
Formal caregivers	1
Former spouse	34
Formulary	139, 143, 207
Full-benefit dual eligible individual	142-143, 151-153, 216-217, 218-219
Full-subsidy eligible (Part D)	151-153, 218-221
Free look	225

G

Gap coverage insurance (drugs)	146, 210
Gatekeeper	20, 61, 183
General (annual) enrollment period	38-40

Generic drugs (Medicare Part D)	140, 146, 153-154, 194, 197, 220-222
Geriatric care manager	1, 15, 125, 246-249
Glaucoma screening	89
Grievance	20, 129, 167-175
Group home (shared housing)	269

H

Health Care Financing Administration (HCFA) (see also Centers for Medicare and Medicaid Services)	32, 224
Health Insurance Portability and Accountability Act (HIPAA)	196, 235-236, 243, 256
Health maintenance organization (HMO)	132, 157, 181, 182-185, 212, 217, 224, 229-232
Hearing aid	50, 66, 70, 161
Hearing before an ALJ	56-57, 176
Heart transplant	67
Hemophilia clotting factors	66
Hemophiliac patient	66
Hepatitis B vaccine	68, 70
High-deductible health policy (HDHP)	162, 196, 197-198, 200, 202, 229
Home and community-based services	28
Home and community-based waiver (long-term care) services	104, 122, 128
Homebound eligibility	27, 41-42, 77, 124, 229

Word Index (WI)
(continued)

Home care agency	2, 4, 8, 10, 12, 22, 54-55, 124
Home care services	1, 7, 13, 17-18, 20, 22, 42, 49, 54-55, 101, 118, 122, 124, 235, 248, 261
Home care worker	3-5, 7-8, 11, 12, 15, 248
Home-delivered meals program (see also Meals on Wheels)	2, 14, 29, 49, 69
Home dialysis	67
Home Equity Conversion Mortgage Insurance Demonstration Act of 1988	251, 253
Home equity conversion plans	2, 251, 258
Home health advance beneficiary notice	54
Home health agency (see also Certified home health agency)	15, 42, 48, 54-55, 77, 83, 177, 247-249
Home health aide	1, 7, 17, 19, 22, 28, 44-45, 49, 124, 248
Home health aide services	18, 44-46, 122-123
Home health care	6, 91
Homebound	2, 14, 24, 27, 31, 41-42, 49, 77, 122, 124, 235, 260
Homemaker services/Home care	1, 28, 46, 50, 52, 267
Homestead	99
Hospice	2, 6, 33, 48, 51-53, 162, 190,

Word Index (WI)
(continued)

	196, 205
Hospital insurance (Medicare Part A)	31-32, 35, 109

I

Immediate annuity	261
Immunizations	70
Immunosuppressive therapy drugs	66
Income (see also Countable income; Earned income; Taxable income; Unearned income)	23, 27, 36, 74-75, 95-96, 98-99, 102-103, 105-114, 117-118, 120, 134, 151-154, 199, 203, 211, 218-222, 235, 245-246, 251, 256, 260, 272, 273
Income cap states (see also 300% state)	107, 108, 113. 114
Income first rule	103
Income spend-down	96
Income-only trust	112, 114, 119-120
Incurred medical expense	107
Indemnity insurance	235
Identification card	32, 95
Independent living retirement community	265-266
Independent review entity (IRE)	32, 167, 168, 173-175, 177-178
Inflation protection	135, 241-242

Word Index (WI)
(continued)

Influenza immunization vaccines	67, 70
Informal caregivers	1, 5, 10, 12
In-home respite care	29
In-home services	6, 13
Initial assessment evaluation (health)	18, 161, 164, 181
Initial coverage limit (Medicare Part D)	145-146, 152, 209-210, 220
Initial determination	32, 56
Initial enrollment period (see also Initial coverage election period)	38-40, 141, 143, 158, 213, 216-217
Injectable drugs	68
In-kind income or support	99
In-patient hospital care	32, 65, 70, 81
Institutionalization	101-102, 104, 119, 238, 267
Institutionalized individual (person)	102, 103, 105, 115, 118, 121. 127
Institutionalized spouse	100-101, 103-106, 108, 111
Instrumental activities of daily living (IADL)	1, 49, 237
Insulin	139, 207
Intensive services	26, 259
Inter vivos trust	111, 114
Intermittent (skilled services)	43-44, 49, 122
Intermittent skilled nursing care	41, 44, 124
Intern and resident services	45, 48
Intraocular lenses	83

Word Index (WI)
(continued)

Intravenous immune gobulin	68
Iron lung	47, 66, 83
Irrevocable trust	111-112, 114, 120

J

Joint assets	99
Joint survivor annuity	261
Judicial review	168, 176

K

Kidney dialysis and transplants (see also End-stage renal disease)	34, 43, 87
Kidneys	67

L

Laboratory services, tests (see also Diagnostic tests)	68, 71, 122, 132
Late enrollment, premium penalty based on	37, 39, 143-144, 216
Laundry	1, 7, 46, 249
Level premium	239
Licensed home care agency	18, 22-23
Licensed practical nurse	19, 43, 45
Lien	127
Life care community	250, 265
Limiting charges (of physician) (see also Charge limit)	91
Liver and lung transplants	67
Living revocable trust	111

Local plan (preferred provider organization)	182, 186-187
Lock-in	183
Long-term care insurance (LTCI)	2, 4, 27, 128, 134-135, 199, 235-246, 251, 256, 258, 260-261, 264
Long-term care ombudsman	29
Long-term care partnership program	134-135
Look-back period	115-118
Low-income Medicare beneficiary	36, 73, 109, 151, 196
Low-income partial subsidy eligibles (Medicare Part D)	151
Low-income premium subsidy	217, 221
Low-income qualifying individuals (QI-1)	75, 110
Low-income subsidy, individual (see also Subsidy-eligible individual)	212, 218, 219, 221

M

Mammogram, mammography	70, 88, 183
Managed care entity/organization	97, 130-133
Managed care plan	189
Mandatory enrollment (Medicaid managed care)	129, 130
Mandatory supplemental benefit	162, 184
Match-up model (shared housing)	269
Maximum approved allowable charge	71, 165
Maximum community spouse resource allowance	104
Meals on wheels	2, 14, 29, 49, 69
Means-tested program	95

Word Index (WI)
(continued)

Medicaid	2, 4-13, 18, 20, 23, 25, 28-30, 36, 61, 73, 92-115, 117-132, 135, 139-142, 146, 149-151, 153, 194, 205-206, 209-210, 212, 215-217, 219, 233, 244-247, 249-251, 256-257, 258
Medicaid dual eligible individual	130, 212
Medicaid managed care	74, 108, 130-132
Medicaid mandatory managed care	128
Medicaid waivers	6, 13, 122
Medical administrative contractor	32
Medical equipment	19, 83, 249
Medical necessity exclusion	70
Medical nutrition therapy	67
Medical Savings Account (MSA)	140, 142, 156-157, 160, 161-163, 165, 179, 184, 196-203, 212, 214
Medical social services	45-47, 52
Medical supplies	19, 45, 47-48, 52, 81, 83, 122
Medically necessary	68, 87, 139, 163, 164, 170, 181, 204, 207, 223, 225, 228, 238
Medically needy	96, 106-107, 113
Medically oriented home care	4, 6, 18, 22, 43,

Word Index (WI)
(continued)

	124, 230
Medicare Advantage	i, 137, 140-141, 155, 158, 160, 162
Medicare Advantage organization	132, 158-160, 164-165, 167-170, 177-178, 184, 207, 212-213, 231-232
Medicare Advantage prescription drug plan (MA-PDP)	140, 142, 148, 159, 207, 209, 212-218
Medicare Advantage program/plan (MAP)	155-166
Medicare Advantage local plan	186-187
Medicare Advantage regional plan	186-187
Medicare application	32, 35, 37-38
Medicare-certified hospice program	51-52
Medicare claim number	32
Medicare eligibility of person 65 or over	35, 39, 63
Medicare enrollment	37-38
Medicare health insurance card	33, 38
Medicare Part A hospital benefits	31-32
Medicare Part B (see Part B)	
Medicare Part C (see Part C)	
Medicare Part D (see Part D)	
Medicare Prescription Drug Improvement and Modernization Act (MMA) (see also Part D)	32, 137-139, 145, 147, 151, 193, 196, 207-208, 211, 216
Medicare prescription drug plan	139, 149, 156, 207-208, 229
Medicare savings programs	148, 152, 211,

	219
Medicare Select	223-224, 229-232
Medicare summary notice	54, 55
Medicare supplemental insurance (see also Medigap)	2, 156, 223, 235
Medicare + Choice (Medicare Part C)	165, 198
Medications	7, 46, 123, 139, 207
Medigap	71, 91, 93, 138, 156, 200, 208, 216, 223-234, 235, 251
Medigap high-deductible policy	223, 229
Mental illness	68, 69, 82
Miller trust	108, 113, 120
Minimum resource allowance (for community spouse)	102, 103-105
Minimum monthly income allowance	102-103
Minimum monthly needs allowance	105
Mobility	1, 239
Monthly basic premium (Medicare Advantage)	161
Monthly premium (for Medicare Part D drugs)	145
Monthly supplemental premium (Medicare Advantage)	161

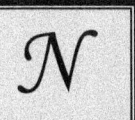

Name-on-the-check rule	108
Naturally occurring retirement community (NORC)	268-269
Network Medicare Advantage Medical Savings Account plan	163
Non-coverage notice	32

Word Index (WI)
(continued)

Non-covered services (exclusions) (Medicare Part B)	69-70
Non-exempt resources, assets	74, 75, 100-102, 109-110
Non-forfeiture clause, protection (LTCI)	239-240, 242-243
Non-formulary drug	139
Non-institutionalized individual	115, 118, 121
Non-medical home care	1, 4, 6-7
Non-network Medical Savings Account plan	199
Non-waivered services	101, 118, 121
Notice of termination of services	58-59
Notice to beneficiary	58
Nursing assessment	125
Nursing care/services	6, 18, 22, 41-43, 52, 66, 69, 95, 101, 102, 123, 236, 249, 262, 265, 266
Nursing facility (home)	1, 24, 27, 61, 77, 84, 87, 104, 105, 107-108, 113, 114, 115, 116, 118, 121, 122, 124, 124, 127, 142, 154, 177, 193, 212, 214, 220, 223, 227, 233, 235, 237, 238, 240, 241, 250, 251, 260, 263, 264
Nursing home without walls	123
Nursing nutritional services	1

Nutritional care counseling	18-19
Nutrition services	6, 29

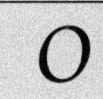

O

Occupational therapist	60, 66, 79-80
Occupational therapy	1, 6, 18-19, 43-44, 52, 66, 77-79, 122
Older Americans Act	2, 13-14, 25, 28-29
Ombudsman	29
Open enrollment period	141, 159-160, 213, 215, 225, 230, 231
Optional categorically needy	106-108
Optional supplemental benefit	184
Optometrist services	70
Organization determination	170-175
Original Medicare	31, 137, 140-141, 155-162, 165, 167, 174, 184, 186, 187, 190, 201, 204-205, 212-2013, 215
Orthopedic shoes	69
Osteoporosis	68
Ostomy care	83, 85
Out-of-pocket costs, expenses, amount, limit	49, 145-146, 152, 156, 185, 187, 209-210, 220, 223, 228,

Word Index (WI)
(continued)

	229, 234
Out-of-pocket threshold (Medicare Part D)	145-146, 153-154, 209-210, 220-222
Outpatient department/hospital services	32, 44, 66, 78, 81, 89, 122
Outpatient mental health services (See also Psychiatric care)	66, 81-82, 227
Outpatient occupational therapy, physical therapy and speech-language pathology	66, 77, 78, 79
Outpatient prescription drugs (Medicare Part D)	138, 140-141, 155, 162, 182, 207-208, 213, 229
Outpatient services (Medicare Part B)	65-66, 69-70
Outpatient skilled therapy	77-79
Oxygen, tents and services	47, 66, 83-85

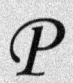

Pacemaker	85
Pap smear screening and pelvic exam	88, 183
Part A (Medicare)	31, 32, 34-39, 51-52, 54, 56, 60, 71, 74-75, 87, 109-110, 137-142, 155-157, 159, 161, 164, 187, 190, 196, 205-207, 213-214, 225, 227, 231
Part B (Medicare)	25, 31-32, 35-40, 44, 54, 56,

Word Index (WI)
(continued)

	60, 64-65, 68-69, 71-79, 81, 82-84, 86-90, 109-110, 137, 139-142, 155-157, 159, 161, 164, 187, 190, 196-197, 205, 207, 212-214, 225, 227-228, 231, 234
Part C (Medicare) (see also Medicare + Choice)	132, 141, 155, 167, 213
Part D (Medicare)	32, 137-147, 149, 151-152, 155-156, 166, 182-183, 186, 190, 192-193, 195, 199, 206-218
Partial hospitalization for mental health treatment	69, 82
Partial subsidy eligible individual	151-153, 218-219, 221-222
Participating provider/physician	72, 185
Part-time or intermittent	44, 122, 124
Partnership program for LTCI	134-135, 246
Pathological services	65
Pelvic examination	88, 183
Period of ineligibility	116-119
Permanent resident alien	35, 38, 96, 98
Permitted deductions	15
Personal care home	263
Personal care (services, aides)	1, 5, 7, 17, 22, 24, 28, 45, 49,

Word Index (WI)
(continued)

	122-125, 228, 230, 235, 244, 249, 256, 263, 265, 266
Personal emergency response system	8, 13
Personal needs allowance	105-106
Physical therapist	65, 79
Physical therapy	6, 18-19, 26, 43-44, 52, 66, 78-79, 122
Physician services	181
Plan of care	6, 7, 20, 41, 42, 45, 47, 48, 52, 78, 79, 125, 244, 250, 256
Plastic surgery	65
Pneumococcal pneumonia vaccine	70
Point of service	157, 184
Pooled trust	113-114, 119-120
Positron emission tomography (PET scan)	90
Poverty level (See Federal poverty level)	
Pre-certification	184
Pre-existing conditions	225-226, 230-232, 242
Pre-existing medical exclusion	159
Preferred provider organization (PPO)	157, 179, 182, 185-187, 224, 229
Premium	35-36, 38, 40, 61, 67, 71-75, 95, 109-110, 137-138, 143-

Word Index (WI)
(continued)

	148, 151-154, 156-157, 161-162, 181, 185, 197, 199-201, 204, 207-211, 215-217, 219-224, 226, 229-231, 235, 238-243, 245, 261
Premium subsidy	154, 217, 219-220
Prescription drugs	47, 69, 93, 137-139, 141-142, 146-147, 149, 151, 153, 155, 161-162, 183, 186, 190, 192, 195, 198-199, 206, 213, 229
Prescription drug plan (PDP)	137-145, 149, 151, 156, 159, 166, 207-218
Preventive care	88-90, 93, 161
Primary care case management	130, 132
Primary care physician	61, 130, 132, 163, 180, 183-184, 190, 192, 205-206
Primary payer	36, 60, 63, 164
Primary plan	60
Private contract (Medicare)	62, 91-92
Private duty nursing	6, 122
Private fee-for-service (PFFS) plan	32, 156-158, 166, 179-180, 204-206, 217

Private room	70
Program for All-Inclusive Care of the Elderly (PACE)	33, 60-61, 106
Prostate cancer screening	88
Prostate-specific antigen (PSA) blood test	86
Protected resource amount	101, 103
Prosthetics (see also Durable medical equipment)	82
Provider-sponsored organization (PSO)	132, 157, 179, 181-182, 189-190
Psychiatric care (see also Mental health care)	68

Q

Qualified disabled and working individual (QDWI)	36, 75, 110, 155, 196, 216
Qualified Individual 1 (see Low-income qualifying individual (QI-1)	
Qualified independent contractor (QIC)	32, 56-57, 59
Qualified Medicare beneficiary (QMB)	74-75, 109-110, 152, 155, 219, 221
Qualifying skilled services (Home care)	41, 43
Qualified medical expenses	197-199, 202, 203
Quality improvement organization (QIO)	32, 58-59, 169

R

Radiation therapy	66
Railroad Retirement benefits	34-35, 37-38, 71, 172, 175
Reasonable and necessary requirement	41-42, 44, 48,

Word Index (WI)
(continued)

	70, 77-78, 84
Reconsideration determination and appeals	58-59, 167-175, 178
Regional preferred provider organization, regional plan	68, 182, 186-188
Rehabilitation (see also Therapy services)	8, 25, 68, 77-78, 82, 259
Religious fraternal benefit (RFB) plan	157, 179, 182, 191-192
Renal dialysis (see also Dialysis)	68, 87, 170
Request for reconsideration	56-57
Residential care facility/home	250, 263
Residential sale leaseback	251
Resources	1, 2, 6, 17, 20, 22-23, 74-75, 95-96, 98-105, 107, 109-111, 117, 127, 134, 137, 147, 151-153, 211, 218-222, 235, 253, 256
Respite care	2, 13, 28, 52, 123,
Reverse mortgage	251-254
Revocable living trust (see also *Inter vivos* trust)	111, 119-120
Risk adjustment payment methodology	195
Robert Wood Johnson program	134, 246
Routine physical examination	70
Rule of deeming	100

S

Seat lift chair	47
Second opinion	65
Secondary payer	33, 36, 60, 64, 164
Section 8 rental subsidy program	271-272
Section 202 program of supportive housing	273-274
Senior center	2, 14-15, 29
Service area	61, 131, 142, 146, 180, 186-187, 192, 214-215
Service termination (see also Termination)	54
Shared housing	268-269
Shelter allowance (see Excess shelter allowance)	
Shoes	69
Shopping	i, 1, 7, 46, 49, 69, 269
Single life annuity	261
Single premium	261
Skilled nursing care	6, 41, 43, 263, 265
Skilled nursing facility	1, 77, 84, 87, 125, 177, 193, 241, 250
Skilled therapy	7, 18, 42, 43-44, 46, 77
Smoking cessation drugs	139, 207
Snapshot day	101-102

Snapshot rule	101-102
Social assessment	125
Social Services and Block Grants	2, 13
Social Security Act	37, 95, 96, 130, 132, 137, 193, 197, 216
Social Security (benefits, income)	12, 32-35, 37-38, 71, 74, 99, 108-109, 113, 161, 175, 273
Social Security Administration (or office)	33, 172, 221
Social welfare agencies and community organizations	24
Social work services	19
Special election period	159-161
Special enrollment period (Original Medicare; Medicare Part D)	39-40, 141-143, 160, 213, 215, 217
Special needs beneficiary, individual	179, 182, 193-194
Special needs trust	112
Special rules for enrolling and disenrolling in an MSA	158
Specialist (physician, care)	61, 90, 163-164, 180-181, 183-184, 192, 205-206
Specialized Medicare Advantage Plans For Special Needs Individuals (SNP)	182, 193-195
Specialty care	163, 181
Specified Low-income Medicare beneficiary (SLMB)	75, 95, 110, 152, 155, 196, 216, 219
Speech-language pathologist	79

Speech-language pathology services (therapy)	43-44, 52, 66, 77, 79
Spend down	96, 98, 106-108, 114
Splint	48, 66, 80-81
Spouse	34, 39, 63, 99-106, 108, 111, 114, 117, 119, 127-128, 199, 202-203, 235, 247, 253-254
Spousal impoverishment	102
Spousal refusal	101, 104, 127
Spousal share	103-105
SSI resource standard	74, 109
SSI states	114
Stand-alone prescription drug plans	137, 140-141, 144, 156, 212-215, 217
Standard coverage determination (Part D)	139, 208
Standard drug plan (Medicare Part D)	145
Standard organization determination	170-171
Standard reconsideration determination	173-174
State partnership programs for LTCI	134, 246
State unit on aging	28
Subluxation	65
Subsidy-eligible individual (see also Low-income subsidy individual)	140, 147, 151, 218
Supplemental needs trust	112
Supplemental Security Income (SSI)	74, 96, 98, 114, 148, 152, 211, 216, 253
Supplementary premium	161, 181

Word Index (WI)
(continued)

Surcharge, premium	39, 71
Surgery	35, 63, 66, 79, 83, 228, 231
Surgical dressings	66
Survivor	35, 128

T

209(b) option	96
300% program	96, 108, 114
Tax advantages (LTCI)	243, 245, 256-257
Taxable income (as relates to MSA)	199, 201-203, 245
Telephone reassurance system	13, 28
Terminally ill	6, 51, 53, 255-256
Termination (services, coverage)	55, 59-59, 129, 131, 166, 170, 177, 215, 232, 240
Testing strips	67
Testamentary trust	111
Therapy services	18, 26, 42, 44, 46, 49, 67, 77-79, 259
Tiered co-payment	146, 210
Time frames (for grievances and appeals)	139, 169-171
Toileting	1, 7, 19, 239, 244
Traditional fee-for-service Medicare, also called Traditional Medicare (see also Original Medicare)	162

Transfer of assets, resources	97, 99, 111-113, 115-121
Transfer penalty	96, 117, 119-121
Transplants/transplantation	66-67
Transportation	13, 24, 25-26, 29, 50, 61, 66, 87, 123, 237, 259, 265, 268
Triggers (LTCI)	238
Trust eligibility rules	111-112
Trust for disabled persons under age 65	112-113
Trust transfer penalty rules	115, 119
Trusts	111-112, 115, 117, 119, 256
Tube feeding	43

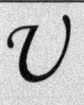

Ultrasound screening	89
Uncompensated value of transferred assets	117, 118
Undue hardship	105, 119
Unearned income	37
Urgent care	183
Utilization review program	158

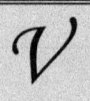

Vaccinations	70
Variable annuity	261-262
Vision care	199-200
Voluntary enrollee	35, 38-39

Word Index (WI)
(continued)

Voucher program (see Section 8 rental subsidy program)	271-272

W

Waiting period	34, 159, 240-242
Waiver programs (see also Medicaid waivers)	6, 13
Waivered home care services	118
Waivered services	121
Walker	7, 24, 47, 83
Welcome to Medicare physical	90
Wheelchairs	24, 47, 66, 83, 85
Wrap-around coverage	63, 93

X

X-rays (see also diagnostic tests)	81

www.ingramcontent.com/pod-product-compliance
Lightning Source LLC
Chambersburg PA
CBHW081125170426
43197CB00017B/2748